MW00439138

The Gastroenterology Resident Pocket Survival Guide

Anil Minocha, M.D., FACP, FACG
Associate Professor of Medicine and Geriatrics

University of Oklahoma and VA Medical Center
Oklahoma City, Oklahoma

International Medical Publishing, Inc.

Other titles from International Medical Publishing:

Clinician's Handbook of Preventive Services, 2nd edition

Guide to Clinical Preventive Services, 2nd edition

The Sixth Report of the Joint National Committee on Prevention, Detection, Evaluation, and Treatment of High Blood Pressure

The Gastroenterology Resident Pocket Survival Guide is provided as an educational resource for physicians. It is not a substitute for supervised training. International Medical Publishing, Inc. and the author provide no warranty for the data or the opinions expressed herein.

First Printing

The Gastroenterology Resident Pocket Survival Guide
A. Minocha, MD, FACP, FACG
International Medical Publishing, Inc.

ISBN 1–883205–39–5

Toll free ordering: 1-800-591-2713
http://www.medicalpublishing.com

Published by International Medical Publishing, Inc.,
P.O. Box 479, McLean, VA 22101-0479

Printed in the United States of America

PREFACE

It's not what we don't know that gets us into trouble. It is what we know that ain't so.

Josh Billings

Digestive conditions account for a large component of a general clinical practice. Put in dollar terms, they contribute to ten percent of health care costs in the US. With the ever expanding and changing field of medicine, it is impossible to know and remember everything at all times, even for the most astute physician, much less a beginner or a general practitioner.

This book intends to provide the reader with basic gastroenterologic information and strategies in an unclouded, abbreviated, and easy-to-read fashion, with the goal of facilitating management of common digestive problems. Towards this end, finer points of grammar have been sacrificed for brevity, and detailed explanations including caveats abandoned to facilitate clarity of concepts. Needless to say that, this book does not propose to be a substitute for the standard text books in medicine or the experience, knowledge, wisdom, and judgement of the consultants.

George Pompiduo, a former French President, said, "Conception is much more fun than delivery." Towards this end, I am deeply indebted to Dr. Thomas Masterson for not only conceiving the idea for this book, but also his ingenious ideas and encouragement throughout this project. Dr. Nathaniel Briggs' patience, perseverance and steadfast efforts have gone a long way in making this a "reader friendly" book. Last but not the least, I owe a deep sense of gratitude to my entire "Minocha family" for their forbearance and endurance with my work-habits throughout this project, as well as, before and after.

As the old saying goes, "I owe my success to the genius of few and dedication of many". This book is dedicated to my loving parents and all of my teachers and mentors throughout my career, who taught me to follow Sir William Osler's teaching, "To prevent disease, to relieve suffering and to heal the sick—this is our work".

Finally, I am reminded of Goethe who said, "It is the process, not the ends we control". An old Chinese proverb states, "Experience is the name one gives to one's past mistakes". I would urge the reader to use this book as a framework for more learning from other bigger sources and asking questions. Please check with your seniors or consultants before trying anything for the first time. Follow Christoph Hufeland, who said, "The physician must generalize the disease and individualize the patient". Towards this latter goal, your easiest and quickest resource is your GI attendings!

CONTENTS

BACKGROUND

ANATOMY AND PHYSIOLOGY
IN GASTROENTEROLOGY

Oropharynx — prepares food for eventual absorption by chewing, stimulation of salivary secretion, and positioning bolus of food for transfer to the esophagus. Saliva contains amylase and lysozyme, enzymes that digest starch and bacteria, respectively. Food bolus is transferred from oropharynx to esophagus by complex neuromuscular mechanisms.

Esophagus — conduit for food from mouth to stomach. Lower esophageal sphincter (LES) prevents reflux of gastric contents into esophagus.

Stomach — secretes gastric juice that contains pepsin, HCl, and gastric lipase. Food mixes with gastric juice secretions, breaks down into small particles, and is slowly released through pylorus into duodenum of small intestine. Pyloric sphincter prevents reflux of duodenal contents.

Small Intestine — stretches from pylorus to ileocecal valve. Most of the digestion and absorption of water and nutrients occurs in the jejunum, except for the absorption of iron, calcium and folic acid that occur mainly in the duodenum. In addition, bile acids and vitamin B_{12} are absorbed in the ileum. Ileocecal valve prevents reflux of colonic contents into the small intestine.

Pancreas — secretes enzymes that digest proteins, fats and carbohydrates. Disorders of the pancreas cause malabsorption syndromes. D-xylose test and small bowel biopsy are normal, while fecal fat excretion test is abnormal. Diseases of small bowel, e.g. celiac sprue and Whipple's disease, have normal digestion but impaired absorption. D-xylose test, fecal fat excretion and small bowel biopsy are abnormal.

Gall Bladder — receives bile from the liver which is delivered to the small intestine during meals. The gall bladder is prone to gallstones when the bile becomes supersaturated with cholesterol.

Colon — most liquid and electrolytes left over from small intestine are absorbed in colon. Colonic bacteria produce gas as a by-product of fermented, unabsorbed carbohydrates. Stool is 75% water, and dead bacteria comprise 30% of solid component of stool.

TYPICAL DAY

GI is generally a consultative service. The attending and fellows typically perform endoscopies in the morning and see patients in the afternoon. The resident serves as the eyes and ears of the service while the attending is busy.

Pre-rounding: See GI inpatients in the morning, especially those patients who had endoscopy the day before, and those being followed for GI bleed.

Check vital signs and perform pertinent abdominal exam on all patients; especially check for distension, tenderness and peritoneal signs. For inpatients with liver disease, pay particular attention to weight, mental status, asterixis, pedal edema, WBC, hematocrit and hemoglobin levels, platelet counts, PT and GI bleed.

See new consults. Organize notes in SOAP format.

Brief attending after seeing the patients. Detailed presentation is done in rounds after endoscopies are finished. Try to review endoscopies on patients you have consulted on.

Rounds: Presentation of new patients is done succinctly, starting with the reason for consultation. Outline non-GI problems followed by description of GI problems, pertinent physical exam findings, problem outline, opinions of other consultants who have seen patient, followed by your assessment and recommendations.

Make decisions on timing of endoscopy or any other procedures, and surgical involvement. Write down orders during or after rounds.

Post-rounds: Schedule tests, write pre-op orders, and call primary care team with your recommendations and plans.

GI HISTORY AND PHYSICAL EXAM

HISTORY

Details and speed of history taking depend on whether the problem is acute, chronic or urgent.

Fever suggests an inflammatory or infectious process (e.g. colitis, Crohn's disease, pancreatitis). Easy fatigability and weight loss may point to chronic diseases such as IBD, TB, cancer, malabsorption syndrome or metabolic disease like DM and thyrotoxicosis. Weight gain suggests functional disorder, fluid overload (e.g. liver cirrhosis, nephrotic syndrome, CHF) or endocrine disease (e.g. Cushing's, hypothyroidism).

Nausea and vomiting are generally nonspecific and occur in a variety of GI and non-GI diseases. They may occur in functional disorders as well as peptic ulcer disease. Vomiting of undigested food consumed a day earlier suggests gastric outlet obstruction or Zenker's diverticulum.

History of heartburn, chest pain, difficulty swallowing, food hanging up in chest, hoarseness, chronic cough, or asthma provide clues to possible gastroesophageal reflux disease.

Dysphagia primarily for liquids occurs in transfer dysphagia (oropharyngeal and neuromuscular disease). Dysphagia for solids implies esophageal obstruction, but may be present in gastric outlet obstruction. Odynophagia is usually caused by infectious, caustic or pill esophagitis, and rarely by reflux esophagitis.

History of abdominal pain in reference to: location, onset, duration, timing (intermittent or constant), quality (sharp, dull, crampy), radiation, precipitating or relieving factors including medications, any accompanying constipation, diarrhea, bloating, or bleeding.

Ask about bowel habits. Be specific: when a patient says "it's okay," this may not really mean "ok" because patients are frequently reluctant to discuss this type of problem. Ask about the number of bowel movements, color, consistency, volume, and odor. Normal patterns vary from 3/day to 3/week. Recent change in bowel habit may be the only presenting symptom of colon cancer.

3

Constipation is defined as two or less bowel movements per week. However, constipation means different things to different people. For example, some have hard, painful stools, and complain of constipation.

Diarrhea is more than 200 g of stool per day. There may be increased fluidity of stool. Increased frequency with stool weight less than 200 g/d is pseudodiarrhea.

Small bowel diarrhea exceeds 1L/d. Osmotic diarrhea resolves on fasting. Acholic stools are light-colored or grayish stools that occur in viral hepatitis and obstructive jaundice.

Many patients without diarrhea have fecal incontinence, but complain of "diarrhea". They may not volunteer information on incontinence unless specifically asked.

Ask about hematemesis or "coffee grounds" emesis. Melena is black, tarry stool usually due to upper GI bleeds, but may also occur from a colonic source. Iron causes black stools that are not tarry and, hence, are heme-negative. Bright, red blood per rectum is usually from an anorectal or sigmoid region, but 5% of severe upper GI bleeds may present with hematochezia.

PHYSICAL EXAMINATION

General exam is important even though focus is on abdominal exam. Duration and details of exam depend upon urgency of situation.

Tachycardia and hypotension call for a quick exam and immediate management. Check texture and color of skin, conjunctivae, nails and sclerae. Look for lymphadenopathy. Spider angiomata, palmar erythema, Dupuytren's contractures and testicular atrophy indicate chronic liver disease.

Inspect abdomen for shape, scars, dilated veins, rash, visible peristalsis or hernia. Bulging flanks indicates ascites.

Auscultate for presence and character of bowel sounds. Listen for at least 2–3 minutes if bowel sounds are absent or infrequent. Frequency is increased in diarrhea. In bowel obstruction, bowel sounds may be high-pitched initially. In pseudo-obstruction, bowel sounds are infrequent and weak or absent. Bruit is heard in arterial narrowing.

Initial palpation is superficial. It relaxes the patient and you can test for tenderness and superficial masses. This is followed by deep palpation. Liver is tender in hepatitis. The healthy spleen is generally not palpable.

Percussion helps in measuring liver/spleen size and detects ascites. Check liver span (normal 6–12 cm) and for any other palpable masses. Rebound tenderness should be initially tested by percussion.

Rebound, involuntary guarding and rigidity suggest peritoneal inflammation.

Shifting dullness and fluid wave indicate ascites.

Pelvic exam in females and rectal exam in all patients is important. Examine for gross and occult blood in stool after rectal exam.

Jaundice is best seen on sclerae, lips, hard palate and skin. Blanching the lips by pressure of glass slide accentuates jaundice. Yellow discoloration of carotenemia is best seen on face, palms and soles.

GI LABORATORY TESTS

LABORATORY TESTS IN GI DISORDERS

GI bleeding: Unexplained anemia suggests occult blood loss from GI tract. Microcytosis suggests iron deficiency anemia. Anemia with high MCV is seen in chronic liver disease, B_{12} deficiency and folate deficiency. Low platelet count and elevated PT/INR suggest liver disease. High BUN favors UGI as a source for GI bleed.

Acute diarrhea: Stools with WBC suggest inflammatory or invasive infectious diarrhea. Order stool tests x 3 for ova and parasites (o+p), culture and sensitivity (c+s), and *Clostridium difficile* toxin to identify the pathogen that is causing the diarrhea.

Chronic diarrhea: Lactose Intolerance — Lactose hydrogen breath test is performed for lactose intolerance. Lactose is ingested and breath is exhaled into a bag every 15–30 minutes. Greater than 20 ppm rise in breath hydrogen indicates lactose intolerance.

Lactulose hydrogen breath is done to look for small bowel bacterial overgrowth, and to measure orocecal transit time. Lactulose is ingested and test performed as in lactose hydrogen breath test. A sharp rise in breath hydrogen within 30–45 minutes suggests small bowel bacterial overgrowth or a rapid small bowel transit.

Check serum gastrin (gastrinoma), calcitonin, VIP (VIPoma), and urinary hydroxyindole acetic acid (carcinoid syndrome) for chronic unexplained diarrhea.

Malabsorption syndrome: 72-hour fecal fat test is performed when patient is ingesting 100 g fat per day. Normal fat excretion is less than 7 g/day. D-xylose is a sugar that does not require digestion prior to absorption. Hence, the test is used to separate maldigestive conditions from mucosal defects of small intestine. 25 g dose of D-xylose is ingested. A one-hour blood sample is taken, and urine is collected for 5 hours. Serum D-xylose < 20 mg/dl or urinary D-xylose < 4 g (16% excretion) suggests impaired intestinal absorptive capacity.

Schilling's test examines the cause for malabsorption of vitamin B_{12}. A small oral dose of radiolabeled B_{12} and a large IM dose of non-radiolabeled B_{12} are administered. Parenterally-administered B_{12} saturates B_{12} binding sites and radiolabeled B_{12} is normally excreted. Less than 8% of radiolabeled B_{12} excretion in 24 hours indicates B_{12} malabsorption. The test is repeated with intrinsic factor administration. If the results are normalized now, it suggests intrinsic factor deficiency. If radiolabeled B_{12} remains abnormal but corrects with administration of pancreatic enzyme supplements, it indicates exocrine pancreatic deficiency. An abnormal test that corrects with administration of antibiotics suggests small bowel bacterial overgrowth.

Liver disease: Low BUN, cholesterol and albumin are seen in liver dysfunction. High SGOT/SGPT suggest liver injury and not liver dysfunction. SGOT/SGPT (SGOT>SGPT) are <500 IU/L in EtOH liver disease. High alkaline phosphatase and GGT suggest intrahepatic or extrahepatic cholestasis. If transaminases and alkaline phosphatase are elevated, the one with a relatively greater increase provides the clue. Elevated ammonia may be present in hepatic encephalopathy, but normal levels do not exclude it.

Pancreatitis: High serum amylase and lipase are seen in pancreatitis. However, high serum amylase may be seen in salivary gland disorders, macroamylasemia, and acute bowel obstruction/perforation/infarction. Serum lipase is elevated in renal failure and acute abdominal conditions. Normal amylase/lipase levels do not exclude pancreatitis. Compared to amylase, lipase has comparable sensitivity but greater specificity. Serum lipase levels are elevated longer than amylase levels.

Viral hepatitis: IgM HAV antibody signifies acute or recent infection with hepatitis A virus (HAV), whereas elevated IgG is seen after acute infection has subsided and suggests immunity to HAV.
HB surface antigen (HBsAg) without HBs antibody indicates acute or chronic HBV infection. Presence of HBs antibody suggests recovery and immunity to HBV. HBV envelope antigen (HBeAg) is seen in highly infectious hepatitis, whereas presence of its HBe antibody suggests decreasing infectivity. Anti-HBV core (anti-HBc) IgM is seen in acute HBV, whereas IgG indicates past infection. Order HBV viral DNA test to confirm presence of virus in blood. Hepatitis D virus antibody indicates acute or chronic HDV infection.

Positive hepatitis C virus (HCV) antibody by ELISA test and confirmed by RIBA test indicates acute ongoing infectivity or past infection. Order HCV RNA by PCR to confirm presence of virus in blood.

Non-viral hepatic disease: 95% of primary biliary cirrhosis cases are positive for anti-mitochondrial antibody (AMA). Low serum copper as well as ceruloplasmin and high urinary copper are seen in Wilson's disease. High ferritin and iron saturation (>50%) are seen in hemochromatosis. Elevated serum ANA, anti-smooth muscle antibody (anti-SMA), anti-liver/kidney microsomal antibody titers, and increased gamma globulins are present in autoimmune hepatitis.

Liver dysfunction: Serum sodium, BUN, albumin, cholesterol are low, while PT is high. Liver enzymes do not correlate with liver dysfunction.

Miscellaneous: High gastrin levels are seen in gastrinoma (Zollinger-Ellison syndrome), pernicious anemia, and proton pump inhibitor therapy (omeprazole and lansoprazole). Normal or elevated CEA levels are seen in cancer of colon and pancreas. Elevated CA 19–9 antigen is seen in 60–75% of pancreatic malignancies.

ERRORS IN MANAGEMENT

COMMON MISTAKES

1. Initial hematocrit in GI bleed is correct. *May take 6–12 hrs to equilibrate; do tilt test.*

2. Dose of sedatives is same in young and elderly, healthy and sick. *Lower dose is required for sedation in elderly and sick patients.*

3. Observe patient with diagnosis of "rule out appendicitis". *All cases of suspected appendicitis should have emergent surgical consultation. A negative Laparotomy rate of 15–20% is acceptable.*

4. Normal endoscopy excludes pathology. *Up to 25% mild esophagitis, 10% gastroduodenal lesions and 5% colon CA are missed during endoscopy.*

5. Endoscopy is always better than barium studies. *Barium swallow with barium pill is superior to endoscopy in detecting subtle esophageal narrowing in patients without odynophagia, bleeding or weight loss.*

6. CT scan is similar to endoscopy. *CT scan is good for solid structures like liver and pancreas, whereas endoscopy visualizes mucosa of luminal gut.*

7. Elevated AST/ALT/alkaline phosphatase abnormal LFTs. *Liver enzymes reflect only injury to the liver and do not correlate with function. Serum albumin, cholesterol and prothrombin time are LFTs.*

8. Peptic ulcer can be diagnosed clinically. *Only a minority of patients with classic "ulcer symptoms" have an ulcer on EGD.*

9. Healing of peptic ulcer makes patients asymptomatic. *Up to 40% with healed ulcers continue to have symptoms.*

10. Normal liver enzymes means normal liver. *Even patients with cirrhosis may have normal liver enzymes.*

11. Markedly elevated liver enzymes in an alcoholic patient are due to alcohol. *Alcoholic liver disease rarely causes transaminase levels to exceed 500 IU/L.*

12. Normal serum pancreatic enzymes exclude pancreatitis. *Serum amylase/lipase may not be elevated in first 24 hours in 10% of cases of acute pancreatitis. Enzymes may be normal in chronic pancreatitis.*

13. One out of 3 guaiac positive cards is indeterminate and warrants fur-

ther guaiac testing. *Patients with polyps/cancer bleed intermittently and even one heme-positive stool warrants further work-up.*

14. Stools are "slightly" guaiac positive. *Either stools are heme-positive or negative; Saying "slightly heme-positive" is like saying "slightly pregnant."*

15. Routine use of FFP and platelet transfusion before paracentesis is indicated in patients with coagulopathy and thrombocytopenia. *Risk of transfusion-related problems is greater than that of developing significant bleed.*

16. Use prophylactic antibiotics for all endoscopic procedures in patients with cardiac problems. *Need for antibiotics depends on type of procedure and the type of underlying medical problem. Antibiotics are not indicated for CABG, pacemakers, ascites, AIDS or prosthetic joints.*

17. Gastritis is a specific clinical entity. *Gastritis means different things to different specialists (e.g. internists, gastroenterologists, pathologists). It also varies according to etiology.*

18. NSAIDs cause injury to stomach only. *NSAIDs can cause injury, including ulcers and strictures, anywhere in GI tract from esophagus to anal canal.*

19. Celiac sprue is a disease of the young. *Up to 25% of cases occur in the elderly.*

20. Follow up of all colon polyps is the same. *In contrast to adenomas, hyperplastic polyps do not have malignant potential. A finding of hyperplastic polyp on flexible sigmoidoscopy does not warrant a colonoscopy or future surveillance.*

21. Use tetracycline for small bowel bacterial overgrowth. *May not respond in up to 60% of cases.*

22. Pill esophagitis occurs in patients with esophageal stricture. *No obvious narrowing of esophageal lumen may be seen on EGD.*

23. Order angiography in patients with ischemic colitis. *Ischemic colitis involves small vessels, and angiography is of no value. Order angiography only if concurrent acute mesenteric ischemia is suspected.*

24. Patients with lactose intolerance need lactose-free diet. *Most lactose intolerant patients can drink up to 240 ml of milk per day.*

25. Patients are put to sleep for endoscopy. *Conscious sedation and not general anesthesia is the rule for most endoscopies in adults.*

26. Use histamine-2 receptor blockers plus sucralfate for peptic ulcer. *Although these two classes of drugs have different mechanism of action, two is not better than one for healing of the ulcer.*

27. Use histamine-2 blockers for peptic ulcer and GERD in similar fashion. *A single nighttime total dose of histamine-2 blocker, e.g. Axid (nizatidine 300 mg), Zantac (ranitidine 300 mg), Pepcid (famotidine 40 mg) is equal in efficacy to twice-a-day split-dosing for peptic ulcer. Twice-a-day split-dosing and not single total nighttime dose, e.g. nizatidine 150 mg bid, ranitidine 150 mg bid, famotidine 20 mg bid is needed in GERD.*

28. Routinely request EGD to exclude penetrating duodenal ulcer as cause of pancreatitis. *Penetrating duodenal ulcer is an extremely rare cause of pancreatitis.*

29. Request colonoscopy to rule out diverticulitis. *Acute diverticulitis is a clinical diagnosis and is managed as such. Colonoscopy is contraindicated in acute diverticulitis especially severe cases. However, colonoscopy should be performed several weeks after resolution of acute episode to exclude malignancy which may be seen in 10% of cases.*

30. Ascribe malabsorption in the elderly to the aging process. *There are no significant changes in absorptive capacity with aging, and malabsorption in the elderly is because of GI disease and not age.*

GI DIAGNOSTIC PROCEDURES

GASTROINTESTINAL IMAGING

PLAIN CXR: Pleural effusion in acute pancreatitis.
- Wide mediastinum or air-fluid level seen in obstructed esophagus.
- Pneumothorax and pneumomediastinum in perforated esophagus.
- Free air under diaphragm indicates perforated abdominal viscus.

ABDOMINAL X-RAY: Air usually in colon and rectum and small amount in small bowel. Air-fluid levels indicate obstruction or ileus. Lack of air in one part of abdomen suggests mass. Irregular lining of the bowel is seen in inflammation, mass or ischemia. Calcification in pancreas suggests chronic pancreatitis.

BARIUM SWALLOW: Rapid sequence esophagram or videoesophagram for transfer dysphagia. Barium swallow with barium pill for obstruction. Benign and malignant strictures can be seen. "Bird beak appearance" is seen in achalasia.

Upper GI X-RAY: Usually done with barium swallow (has to be ordered separately). Visualizes mid-esophagus to distal duodenum. Good for ulcers and tumors, but less accurate than endoscopy.

SMALL BOWEL X-RAY: Need to order separately from UGI X-ray. Visualizes entire small bowel. Mass lesions, strictures and fistulae can be seen.

SMALL BOWEL ENTEROCLYSIS: Barium is injected via a tube into the duodenum. Small amount of barium used, so loops of bowel are better visualized. More accurate than small bowel series but more cumbersome.

BARIUM ENEMA: Air-contrast barium enema better than barium alone. Not good for rectosigmoid region; flexible sigmoidoscopy is warranted.

ORAL CHOLECYSTOGRAM: Accuracy is similar to ultrasound, so not used much these days. Radiopaque dye is ingested. Ineffective if serum bilirubin >3 mg/dl.

INTRAVENOUS CHOLANGIOGRAPHY: Both gall bladder and bile ducts are visualized. Visualization of bile ducts is poor, so out of favor.

PERCUTANEOUS TRANSHEPATIC CHOLANGIOGRAPHY (PTC): Performed to visualize bile ducts. Successful in 90% of cases with dilated bile ducts. High failure rate in normal bile ducts. Usually used if ERCP fails or is unavailable. Catheter can be placed for drainage in biliary obstruction.

CT SCAN: Good for solid organs, not for bowel wall.

- Better than ultrasound for pancreas (ultrasound better for bile ducts).
- Better than liver-spleen scan for focal hepatic lesions.
- CT-guided aspiration and biopsy of lesions can be performed.

ULTRASOUND: Less expensive than CT; can be done as portable.

- Good for gallstones and measuring bile duct size.

ANGIOGRAPHY: Can localize site of bleeding or occlusion in vessels.

- Bleeding rate should be at least 0.5 ml/min for localization.
- Can perform therapeutic embolization.
- Can administer intra-arterial vasopressin to stop bleeding, papaverine in ischemic bowel and chemotherapy for cancer.

LIVER-SPLEEN SCAN: Functional and anatomic test for liver. CT is better for focal lesions. Colloid shift (ribs, spine are seen) suggests liver disease.

HIDA SCAN: Nonvisualization of gall bladder indicates acute cholecystitis.

- Not good for bile ducts.

LABELED RBC SCAN: Used to localize site of intermittent bleeding.

- Minimum rate of bleeding should be 0.1 ml/min.
- Also used for diagnosis of hepatic hemangioma.

ABDOMINAL MRI: Useful in diagnosis of hepatic hemangioma and small intra-abdominal lesions not detected by CT.

UPPER and LOWER ENDOSCOPY

Esophagogastroduodenoscopy

Visualization of esophagus, stomach and proximal duodenum. Can take biopsies, cauterize bleeding lesions and perform sclerotherapy or band ligation of varices. PEG feeding tube can be placed.

Except in emergency, EGD usually done after 6-hour fast. Most patients are given local anesthetic spray to oropharynx and IV sedation.

Indications: dyspepsia refractory to conventional treatment, upper GI bleed, dysphagia and odynophagia, caustic ingestion, meat impaction, and eradication of esophageal varices in patients with history of variceal bleed.

Contraindications: suspected perforation of viscus, combative and unstable patients.

Complications: bleeding, perforation, respiratory problems and arrhythmias.

Flexible sigmoidoscopy

Visualization of distal colon and rectum with short (65 mm) scope. Indicated for hematochezia, and colon cancer screening in asymptomatic average-risk patients >50 yrs. Cleansing enema (see page 24) used just prior to exam. Sedation usually not used.

Colonoscopy

Visualization of entire colon and scope the terminal ileum. Variety of cleansing regimens requiring 1–3 days of bowel prep. Oral Fleet Phospho soda or polyethylene glycol (PEG) are commonly used (see page 24). IV sedation used. Biopsies, polypectomy and electrocautery can be done.

Indications: altered bowel habit, unexplained diarrhea or abdominal pain, heme-positive stools, lower GI bleed, inflammatory bowel disease, colonic polyps or unexplained iron deficiency anemia.

Contraindications: perforated viscus, severe colitis or diverticulitis, and unstable patient.

ENDOSCOPIC RETROGRADE CHOLANGIOPANCREATOGRAPHY (ERCP)

NPO after midnight. Check CBC, PT and PTT.

Many endoscopists use some kind of antibiotic.

Pre-op antibiotic (ceftriaxone 2 g IV). Instead of IV antibiotics, gentamicin 80 mg mixed in 50 ml of radiopaque dye may be used as contrast.

Radiopaque contrast injected into bile and pancreatic ducts, and ducts are visualized under fluoroscopy. Mucosal biopsies, brushing for cytology, sphincterotomy, stent placement and stone retrieval from duct can be done.

Indications: extrahepatic obstruction of biliary system, pancreatic mass and recurrent pancreatitis of unknown etiology, suspected primary sclerosing cholangitis.

Complications: similar to EGD. Significant risk for pancreatitis. After ERCP, transient asymptomatic elevation of pancreatic enzymes occurs. Do not check pancreatic enzymes in the absence of symptoms and signs.

LIVER BIOPSY

Indications: unexplained liver abnormalities, assessment of histology for chronic HBV or HCV, suspected malignancy, hemochromatosis, Wilson's disease, sarcoidosis.

Outpatient procedure: ability to cooperate is important.
Biopsy done blind or can be guided by ultrasound or CT.

NPO after midnight. Usually done in AM so patient can be monitored for 5–8 hours before discharge.

Check Hgb, platelets, PT, recent ultrasound or CT to image liver.

Contraindications: uncooperative patient, PT >3 sec above control, platelets <50 k/mm^3, infected pleural effusion, peritonitis, and massive ascites.

Complications: bleeding, pneumothorax. Check Hgb, CXR; may need chest tube for pneumothorax.

CONSCIOUS SEDATION

Benzodiazepines and opiates are the most commonly used classes of medication. Frequently they are combined. Midazolam (Versed) is used more than diazepam (Valium). Diazepam is long-acting with more side effects. Meperidine (Demerol) is the most frequently used opiate. Its dose, sufficient to produce apnea and analgesia, may not be sufficient to induce sleep. Sedation is usually started with meperidine 50 mg IV and midazolam 1 mg IV. Half of both drugs, or only one drug, is used in elderly or very sick patients.

Haloperidol is effective in agitated patients especially alcoholics.

Meperidine, fentanyl and haloperidol are FDA Category C. Midazolam is FDA Category D. Diazepam is not recommended at all during pregnancy. Midazolam, propofol, fentanyl and haloperidol are excreted in human milk.

Serious complications are rare and mostly cardiopulmonary.

Monitoring of vital signs and continuous pulse oximetry is mandatory.

Post-procedure monitoring generally ranges from 30–120 minutes.

Naloxone (0.4 mg IV initially) and flumazenil (Romazicon 0.2 to 1 mg) are specific antagonists of opiates and benzodiazepines, respectively.

ANTIBIOTIC PROPHYLAXIS

Not used for routine EGD and colonoscopy. Antibiotics prophylaxis is indicated for esophageal dilatation and variceal sclerotherapy in patients with prosthetic valves, h/o endocarditis, systemic-pulmonary shunts and new synthetic vascular graft (<1 year old).

Patients with CABG, pacemakers, ascites, AIDS or prosthetic joints don't require prophylaxis.

Ampicillin 2 g and gentamicin 80 mg IV 30 minutes before endoscopy and amoxicillin 1.5 g po 6 hours after the procedure. Vancomycin 1 g IV plus gentamicin is used in penicillin-allergic patient.

In low-risk patients, amoxicillin 3 g po (with sip of water) 1 hr before and 1.5 g po 6 hours after the procedure.

Antibiotics are recommended for all patients prior to PEG placement (cefazolin 1g IV) and for ERCP in cases of suspected biliary tree obstruction and pancreatic pseudocyst.

GASTROINTESTINAL PHARMACOTHERAPEUTICS

GASTROINTESTINAL DRUGS

ANTACIDS

Sodium bicarbonate effective in neutralizing acid but followed by acid rebound. Side effects: alkalosis, gas, increased sodium load. Not preferred.

Aluminum and magnesium containing antacids are effective in healing ulcers. Aluminum oxide causes no acid rebound. Side effect is constipation. Magnesium oxide causes diarrhea and is usually combined with aluminum antacids.

Calcium antacids cause milk-alkali syndrome and rebound acid secretion.

HISTAMINE-2 RECEPTOR ANTAGONISTS

Cimetidine (Tagamet 800 mg) is clinically equivalent to 300 mg of ranitidine (Zantac) or nizatidine (Axid) and 40 mg of famotidine (Pepcid). Single nighttime dose is effective for duodenal ulcer. Taking histamine-2 receptor blockers and antacids together may decrease histamine-2 receptor blocker absorption.

Cimetidine, and less so ranitidine, have drug interactions by inhibition of cytochrome P_{450} system. Cimetidine increases blood levels of theophylline, warfarin and phenytoin.
Cimetidine side effects: headache, GI upset, impotence, gynecomastia, and altered mental status.
Nizatidine side effects: sweating, urticaria, and somnolence.

PROTON PUMP INHIBITORS (PPIs)

Lansoprazole (Prevacid) 30 mg po qd and Omeprazole (Prilosec) 20 mg qd .
Higher doses needed in refractory ulcers and severe gastroesophageal reflux disease.

Lansoprazole 30 mg po qd produces a significantly longer duration of increased intragastric pH level as well as faster symptomatic relief when compared with omeprazole 20 mg po qd. The two drugs are equally effective in raising intragastric pH in *H. pylori*-negative subjects, and overall healing rates are equivalent.

19

Side effects: minimal. Check for drug interactions as in histamine-2 receptor blocker. Lansoprazole is FDA Category B and omeprazole is Category C for use in pregnancy.

MUCOSAL PROTECTIVE AGENT

Sucralfate (Carafate 1 g po qid) heals ulcers by its local effects without affecting acid secretion. Also used as slurry for pill esophagitis.

PROSTAGLANDIN ANALOGS

Misoprostol (Cytotec): antisecretory and mucosal protective agent. 200 mcg po qid with food prevents NSAID-induced ulcers. Side effects: abdominal pain and diarrhea.

PROKINETICS

Indications: gastroparesis, gastroesophageal reflux disease, non-ulcer dyspepsia, pseudo-obstruction, and constipation.

Metoclopramide (Reglan 10–20 mg po qid or 10 mg IV). Side effects: mild anxiety, dystonia, tardive dyskinesia.
Cisapride (Propulsid 10–20 mg po qid). Side effect: diarrhea (no CNS toxicity). Cardiac arrhythmias if used with erythromycin, ketoconazole, itraconazole, nefazodone, clarithromycin, fluconazole, indinavir, ritonavir, phenothiazines, tricyclic and tetracyclic antidepressants, quinidine, procainamide, astemizole, bepridil, sparfloxacin or terodiline. Also contraindicated in patients with history of prolonged QT interval, ventricular arrhythmias, renal failure, CHF.

During acute episode of gastroparesis: erythromycin 3 mg/kg IV q 8 hours x 5–7 days. Then discontinue erythromycin and start cisapride.

ANTIEMETICS

Dimenhydrinate (Dramamine) 50 mg po tid; meclizine 25 mg po tid.
Prochlorperazine: tranquilizer and antiemetic.

Ondansetron (Zofran), granisetron (Kytril), dolasetron (Anzemet): Potent agents for chemotherapy-induced emesis. Side effects: typically limited to headache, constipation, diarrhea.

Ondansetron: 16–32 mg IV for chemotherapy-induced and 4 mg IV or 8 mg po q 12 hours for post-op nausea/vomiting.
Granisetron: 10 mcg/kg IV before chemotherapy or 1 mg po bid on day

of chemotherapy, and each day chemotherapy is given.

Dolasetron: 100 mg IV before chemotherapy, and 12.5 mg IV for post-operative cases.

Tetrahydrocannabinol in marijuana is effective for chemotherapy-induced emesis. THC is available as Dronabinol (5–10 mg po q 4–6h). Side effects: dryness of mouth, drowsiness and orthostatic hypotension.

AMINOSALICYLATES

Sulfasalazine (2–4 g/d) is the prototype. Aminosalicylate is active moiety, although most toxicity is related to sulfa component. Drink plenty of water. Side effects: headache, GI upset, reversible hypospermia, pancreatitis, hepatitis, colitis.

Mesalamine and olsalazine have no sulfa moiety and are less toxic. Potential for nephrotoxicity with mesalamine.

Asacol (oral mesalamine 1.6–4.8 g/d po) releases 5–ASA at pH of 7 or above, corresponding to that of the terminal ileum. Pentasa (oral mesalamine 4 g/d po) contains microspheres that release drug throughout GI tract.

Mesalamine (Rowasa) enema 4 g qhs *or* mesalamine supp 500 mg bid for intra-rectal administration.

Olsalazine (Dipentum 0.75–1.5 g/d) consists of two 5–ASA molecules joined by a bond that is broken down by colonic bacteria, releasing 5–ASA. Diarrhea is common.

CORTICOSTEROIDS

For IV, po, and intra-rectal administration.

Indications: IBD, autoimmune hepatitis, post-transplant, GVHD, severe alcoholic hepatitis.

Side effects: muscle breakdown, immunosuppression, osteoporosis, hyperglycemia, delayed wound healing, opportunistic infections, body habitus changes, hirsutism, hypertension.

Prescribe exercise, calcium and vitamin D to preserve skeletal tissue.

IMMUNOSUPPRESSIVES

Azathioprine (Imuran) breaks down to 6-mercaptopurine (6-MP) in the body. Used for patients requiring long-term steroids (e.g. IBD, autoimmune hepatitis), 50–150 mg/d po helps in reducing the dose of steroids and their long-term side effects.

Side effects: hepatotoxicity, bone marrow suppression (monitor CBC), and pancreatitis. Risk for neoplasms not proven in IBD.

Cyclosporine is used in toxic megacolon due to ulcerative colitis (4 mg/kg/d IV infusion), inflammatory and fistulous Crohn's disease (4 mg/kg/d IV infusion, or 5–7.5 mg/kg/d po), as well as in liver transplant cases to prevent rejection. Dose-related nephrotoxicity occurs. Monitor drug levels.

LAXATIVES

Bulk laxatives: Limited role in chronic constipation. Use with plenty of water.
Psyllium (Metamucil): moist soft stool. Side effect: bloating.
Methylcellulose (Citrucel 1 tbsf bid to tid).

Lubricant laxatives: Mineral oil 15 ml. Prevents absorption of fat-soluble vitamins. Contraindicated in the elderly or in dementia.

Saline cathartics: Act by increasing osmotic pressure.
Milk of Magnesia (magnesium hydroxide): 30–60 ml; use lower dose in concentrated formulations.
Magnesium citrate 6–12 oz po: Avoid in diabetes because of high sugar content, and in renal failure.

Irritant laxative: Dulcolax tabs or suppository. Dose 10 mg.

Stool softeners: Do not increase bulk or irritate gut. Pericolace 1–2 cap qd.

BILE ACID (URSODEOXYCHOLIC ACID)

Ursodiol (Actigall) improves abnormal liver function in cholestatic diseases like primary biliary cirrhosis and primary sclerosing cholangitis. Used in selected cases of uncomplicated gallstone disease and idiopathic recurrent pancreatitis.
Dose: 8–15 mg/kg/d. No side effects.

ANTIVIRAL AGENTS

Ganciclovir for CMV: 5 mg/kg IV q 12 hour x 2–4 wks, followed by maintenance treatment (1 g po tid with food) in immunosuppressed patients.
Foscarnet for CMV: 60 mg/kg q 8 h or 90 mg/kg IV q 12 h x 2–4 wks followed by maintenance treatment (90–120 mg/kg/d IV infusion over 2 h individualized for renal function).
Foscarnet for acyclovir-resistant HSV: 40 mg/kg IV q 8–12 h x 2–3 wks followed by maintenance of 90 mg/kg/d IV over 2 h in immunosuppressed.

Acyclovir for herpes simplex esophagitis (5 mg/kg IV over 1 h q 8 h x 7–10 d) followed by oral HSV prophylaxis (400 mg po bid) in immunosuppressed. Acyclovir is not for CMV infection.

Alfa-interferon (Intron A, Roferon-A) is indicated in HBV and HCV infection.

Dose 3 million units s.c. q 3 times per wk for 12 months in hepatitis C in patients who respond, and 5 million units s.c. qd for 16 wks for hepatitis B.

Side effects include initial flu-like reaction (fever, headache, malaise). Chronic side effects include fatigue, depression and bone marrow suppression. Monitor CBC q wk x 4, then q 2 wks x 4, then monthly.

Ribavirin plus interferon (Rebetron) is used in HCV in fresh cases as well as nonresponders or those who relapse after treatment with interferon alone. Monitor Hgb because of hemolytic anemia due to Ribavarin.

Interferon alfacon-1 (Infergen) is a synthetic interferon. Dose 9 mcg s.c. three times per wk. If no response in 12 wks, increase dose to 15 mcg s.c. three times per wk.

Interferon is contraindicated if platelet count <100,000/ml or leukopenia <3000 cells/ml. Some use reduced dose of interferon for platelet count between 50K–100K/mm^3.

ANTIBACTERIAL

Metronidazole (Flagyl): used in abdominal infections (500 mg IV q 6 h), amebiasis. (750 mg tid x 10 d), Crohn's disease (250 mg tid to 500 mg qid) and pseudomembranous colitis (250–500 mg po tid). Side effects: GI upset, metallic taste, neuropathy.

BILE ACID BINDING AGENT

Cholestyramine (Questran) is a resin that binds to bile acids preventing reabsorption. Used for C. difficile colitis, pruritus and bile salt diarrhea.

Side effects: constipation, bloating. Maximum of 16 g/d in divided doses. Other medications should be taken at least 2 hours apart.

SOMATOSTATIN ANALOG

Octreotide is useful for variceal hemorrhage (50–100 mcg IV bolus and 50 mcg/h infusion). For severe IBS and severe dumping syndrome, give 25–50 mcg q ac.

ANTI-TUMOR NECROSIS FACTOR

Infliximab (Remicade) is a monoclonal antibody against tumor necrosis factor-alpha.

It is given as a single IV infusion of 5 mg/kg over 2 hours for moderate to severely active Crohn's disease unresponsive to conventional treatment. In cases of fistulizing Crohn's disease, the initial dose is repeated at 2 wks and 6 wks.

Side effects: infections, lupus-like syndrome, infusion-related reaction, GI upset.

PREPARATION FOR FLEXIBLE SIGMOIDOSCOPY

Fleet enema x 1–2, one to two hours before procedure. Some add magnesium citrate 10 oz po the night before.

PREPARATIONS FOR COLONOSCOPY

Fleet Phospho soda preparation: two 1.5 oz. bottles OTC

At noon, mix one 1.5 ounce bottle of Fleet Phospho soda with 4 oz. of cool water and drink; follow with 8 oz. glass of clear liquid. Repeat with second Fleet Phospho soda in evening. Drink 3–4 more glasses of water before going to bed. Caution in renal insufficiency.

PEG solution protocol (CoLyte or GoLytely available by prescription only)

Solution made just before use. Add water to fill the container.

Start at 3:00 PM and drink the entire gallon over 3–4 hrs.

For difficult to cleanse patients, order a 10 oz. oral magnesium citrate (OTC) at 1:00 PM.

GASTROINTESTINAL SYNDROMES
NAUSEA AND VOMITING

Nausea is a sensation, whereas vomiting is a well-coordinated motor act. Nausea is frequently but not always associated with vomiting. Regurgitation occurs when esophagogastric contents come up into the oropharynx without the neuromuscular activity seen in vomiting.

The first step in assessment is to determine whether symptoms are acute or chronic. Associated symptoms and signs, and relationship with meals provide clues to diagnosis.

Postprandial vomiting is seen in gastric outlet obstruction due to ulcer or cancer. Patients with benign obstruction are usually hungry, whereas cancer leads to anorexia and weight loss. Regurgitation of undigested food is seen in achalasia.

Acute fever suggests an infectious etiology. When associated with mental status changes, nausea and vomiting implies a CNS lesion, whereas abdominal pain and diarrhea suggest gastroenteritis.

Drugs causing nausea and vomiting include erythromycin, chemotherapeutic agents, and digoxin. Projectile vomiting is seen with elevated intracranial pressure (do fundoscopy).

Physical exam should include vital signs and a tilt test to assess volume status; abdominal exam for bowel sounds (high-pitched in bowel obstruction, absent in ileus), tenderness (ulcer, cholecystitis, pancreatitis), peritoneal signs (peritonitis), and succussion splash (gastroparesis and outlet obstruction).

Work-up: includes chemical profile, CBC, serum amylase/lipase, flat and upright abdominal films. High WBC is seen in infectious/inflammatory processes. RUQ ultrasound and HIDA scan with CCK ejection are helpful for hepatobiliary-pancreatic lesions.

Treatment of nausea and vomiting depends on the cause.

Gastroparesis: cisapride (Propulsid 10–20 mg qid), metoclopramide (10–20 mg po qid).

Chemotherapy-induced: ondansetron 16–32 mg IV before chemotherapy, granisetron, dolasetron, phenothiazines, benzodiazepines (lorazepam), cannabinoids and steroids.

Post-op: ondansetron (Zofran) 4 mg IV or 8 mg po qbid; dolasetron 12.5 mg IV; granisetron (Kytril) 10 mcg/kg IV qd or 1 mg po bid.

Motion sickness: scopolamine, promethazine, and meclizine.
Vestibular disease: antihistamines (e.g. promethazine or meclizine).
Drug/radiation-induced: prochlorperazine or chlorpromazine.

ACUTE ABDOMINAL PAIN

Do quick history and physical to decide if patient needs emergent surgery. Do not give analgesics or sedatives until assessment is made.

Ask about onset, duration, character, location, severity, and radiation of pain, associated symptoms, aggravating/remitting factors, as well as co-morbid conditions. Pulmonary, cardiac and back problems may present as abdominal pain. In addition, gynecologic and obstetric problems may present as abdominal pain in females.

Pain of perforated peptic ulcer or ruptured aortic aneurysm, spontaneous pneumothorax, and bowel infarction are sudden in onset. Colicky pain occurs due to some obstruction (bowel, ureteral or biliary), is rapid in onset, and pain gets better between attacks. Pain due to an inflammatory or infectious process (appendicitis, pancreatitis, or cholecystitis) may be rapid or gradual in onset and peaks over several hours.

Location of pain provides helpful clues, e.g. right subscapular pain (biliary or hepatic source), epigastric (stomach or colon), RUQ pain (hepatobiliary or gastroduodenal), flank pain (kidney), hypogastrium (colon or kidney), groin/genitalia (ureter or bladder), and umbilicus (appendicitis).

Patient with shallow breathing, lying still with flexed hips, suggests peritonitis. Patients with colic are usually thrashing about. Pale, shocky patient on anticoagulants suggests intra-abdominal hemorrhage. Fever with tachycardia, hypotension, diaphoresis is possibly a surgical abdomen.

Check for visible peristalsis in cases of suspected obstruction and strangulation. Decreased or absent bowel sounds are usually seen in ileus. Normal bowel sounds don't exclude surgical abdomen. Intestinal obstruction initially leads to hyperactive bowel sounds. Presence of tenderness, rebound, guarding, and rigidity suggest peritonitis.

Testing for rebound by deep tenderness and rapid release is uncomfortable for patient and not reproducible. Percussion tenderness is a gentler method of testing for rebound. Extension of the thigh at the hip (psoas sign) and internal rotation of the thigh with knee flexed (obturator sign) elicit pain in appendicitis.

Rectal and pelvic exam may point to appendicitis, pelvic inflammatory disease (PID), twisted ovarian cyst or ectopic pregnancy.

Work-up: CBC – high WBC suggests infection/inflammation; falling platelet count suggests sepsis or DIC; dropping Hgb level implies bleeding or hemolysis; UA, routine chemistries, serum amylase/lipase, human beta-chorionic gonadotropin (HCG) in women, EKG.
Flat and upright abdominal X-ray as well as PA and lateral views of chest must be done. If patient can't stand upright, get left lateral decubitus to exclude free air in the peritoneum.

Ultrasound is simple, non-invasive and useful for visualizing the biliary system, pancreas, abdominal aorta and pelvic organs in females. CT is helpful for solid organs like the pancreas, and to exclude abscess. Angiography may be diagnostic as well as therapeutic for patients with acute mesenteric ischemia.

Acute pancreatitis: common in alcoholics or patients with gallstones. Serum amylase may be elevated in perforated or strangulated bowel.

Acute appendicitis: pain in midline and then RLQ; fever, RLQ tenderness and leukocytosis with left shift. Pain worsened by movement or coughing. RLQ ultrasound may help. Abdominal spiral CT is most helpful. Differential diagnosis includes mesenteric lymphadenitis, diverticulitis and PID. Treatment is surgical. A negative laparotomy rate of 15–20% is acceptable.

Acute gastroenteritis: diffuse abdominal cramps and tenderness with nausea, vomiting, and diarrhea.

Acute cholecystitis: severe epigastric or RUQ pain with nausea and vomiting, fever and RUQ tenderness, leukocytosis, mild hyperbilirubinemia and abnormal liver enzymes. Ultrasound shows gallstones. Non-visualization of gall bladder on HIDA scan.

Acute diverticulitis: LLQ pain, fever, tenderness, leukocytosis.

Acute intestinal obstruction: crampy pain, vomiting, abdominal distension, hyperperistalsis and distended bowel. Air-fluid levels present on upright abdominal X-ray.

Perforated viscus: sudden onset of abdominal pain, distention, and free air under diaphragm.

Acute mesenteric ischemia: abdominal pain out of proportion to clinical findings, bloody diarrhea, leukocytosis and lactic acidosis in patient with history of CHF, arrhythmias, hypotension, peripheral vascular disease, or birth control pills. Diagnosis is by selective mesenteric angiography.

Acute superior mesenteric artery thrombosis occurs at site of atherosclerosis. Embolic occlusion occurs due to left atrial or ventricular thrombus. Treatment is preoperative papaverine via angiography catheter (30–60 mg/h) and surgery.

Chronic thrombosis and minor emboli without peritoneal signs are managed medically.
Non-occlusive mesenteric ischemia is usually preceded by a cardiovascular event. Treatment: papaverine infusion. If peritoneal signs are present, treatment is surgery.

Mesenteric venous thrombosis occurs in hypercoagulable states, e.g. protein C and S deficiency, birth control pills, and in leukemias. CT can identify a lesion in 90%. If CT is negative, angiography should be done. Treatment is with anticoagulant or thrombolytic therapy. Surgery is required if signs of bowel infarction are present.

ACUTE GASTROINTESTINAL BLEEDING

Management of an unstable patient more important than looking for cause of bleed.

Normal vital signs with tilt positive (fall of BP by 10 mm or increase in pulse ≥20/min) indicate 5–20% of volume depletion. Hypotension, impaired mentation, tachycardia, oliguria (<30 ml/hr) indicate severe blood loss (>40%).

Initially, Hct and Hgb levels may be normal, even in severe bleeding. Approximately 85–90% of bleeds cease spontaneously. Record color of stool for monitoring. Bright red blood per rectum in upper GI bleed suggests severe ongoing blood loss.

Secure IV access (at least 2) with large bore IV catheter. Obtain blood for CBC, PT, SMAC, type and cross-match at least 4 units packed red blood cells (PRBC).

Rapid IV saline infusion; in hypotensive patients, administer PRBC as soon as cross-matched blood is available. In severe emergencies, type-specific blood (type O) may have to be given. Patients requiring massive transfusion should preferably receive warmed blood. Hgb rises by 1 gram for each unit of PRBC.

Give one unit of fresh frozen plasma (FFP) for every 4 units of PRBC for patients with normal PT/PTT. If patient has coagulopathy, higher doses of FFP are needed. Give platelet infusion for platelet count <50,000. Calcium gluconate may be needed in case of massive transfusion.

Vasopressors are not helpful since the problem is volume loss. Insert NG tube. In case of obvious upper GI bleed, it helps to assess rate of blood loss. In case of unclear source, it helps in localizing source of the bleed. 5% of severe hematochezia is due to upper GI bleeds. Patients with acute, severe upper GI bleed may need to be intubated, especially before endoscopy, to protect airway from aspiration.

Admit to ICU and monitor vital signs, urine output, mental status, CBC, and electrolytes.

Detailed history: Performed after initial assessment and resuscitation when patient is stable. Ask about abdominal pain and previous history of bleed. Patients with peptic ulcer, esophagitis, esophageal tumors, bowel ischemia and inflammatory bowel disease may provide history of abdominal pain. Bleeding is painless in varices, AVM's, diverticulosis, and hemorrhoids.

Previous history of a bleed may provide clue to a source of the present bleed.
History of alcohol use: alcohol can cause bleeding by Mallory-Weiss tear of mucosa during alcohol-induced vomiting/retching, and through liver disease and portal hypertension. Source of bleed in patients with prior h/o variceal bleed may not be varices in 40–50% cases.
History of chronic liver or kidney disease, abdominal aortic aneurysm repair.
History of medications: NSAIDs and methotrexate cause GI ulceration; antiplatelet drugs and coumadin promote bleeding.

Exam: In addition to vital signs and mental status, check for stigmata of chronic liver disease (jaundice, palmar erythema, spider nevi, ascites), skin for possible bleeding diathesis (ecchymoses and petechiae), nose and throat for trauma, tumors, and abdomen for hepatosplenomegaly, tenderness, ascites. Perform rectal exam for stool color, consistency and volume.

Upper GI bleeding
Etiology: ulcer (45%), erosions (25%) and varices (10%).

Mortality high in elderly and patients with varices or gastric cancer.

False negative NG aspirate occurs in 15% cases.

Treatment: IV fluids, histamine-2 receptor blockers. PRBC, FFP and vitamin K as needed. Octreotide infusion (50–100 mcg bolus and 50 mcg/h) in suspected varices.

Urgent EGD indicated for patients with bleeding varices, bleeding that does not stop, or bleeding that restarts shortly after ceasing.

Ulcer with a clean base rebleeds in 1% of cases, whereas one with a visible vessel may rebleed in 50%. Therapeutic EGD helps in reducing rebleeding and the need for surgery.

Sclerotherapy or banding of esophageal varices is performed to stop bleeding and to prevent recurrence. Octreotide is the drug of choice for bleeding varices (start asap).

Vasopressin/nitroglycerin IV infusion is toxic and effective in only 50%. Balloon tamponade if bleeding does not stop despite above treatment. Consider transjugular intrahepatic portosystemic shunt (TIPS) for patients refractory to above measures.

Sclerotherapy or banding also done to eradicate esophageal varices and prevent recurrence of bleeding. It is not effective in preventing gastric variceal hemorrhage. Propranolol (20–40 mg po bid to reduce heart rate by 25%) and nadolol are effective in preventing initial as well as recurrent variceal hemorrhage.

Lower GI bleed

Five percent of severe hematochezia may be due to upper GI source. Insert NG tube to look for blood. Biliary aspirate excludes active upper GI bleed. Clear, nonbilious aspirate excludes bleed proximal to pylorus (false negative occurs in 15%).

Upper GI bleed manifesting as hematochezia is accompanied by hemodynamic instability. Melena may occur from a colonic source.

Painless lower GI bleed: diverticulosis, AVM, hemorrhoids, neoplasia. Painful lower GI bleed: colitis, IBD, infections, or ischemia.

Diverticulosis causes massive painless bleed. Amount and severity of bleeding variable in AVM and neoplasia. Bright, red blood only on toilet paper or streaking on stool reflects anorectal source.

Flexible sigmoidoscopy (Flex sig) or, preferably, a colonoscopy is the test of choice to localize source of bleed. If patient is stable, prepare the colon for colonoscopy using standard prep. If nondiagnostic, order 24-hour RBC bleeding scan in case of intermittent bleed (>0.1 ml/min).

Order angiogram if there is an active bleed (1–2 ml/min). Intra-arterial vasopressin or selective embolization can be done during angiography. Consider surgery in life-threatening cases.

DIARRHEA

There is a wide range of normal bowel movement patterns, from 3/d to 3/wk. Diarrhea is an increase in frequency, amount, volume or fluidity of stool. Normal is <200 g/d of stool.

Ask for frequency, consistency, volume and duration. Be specific about urgency, incontinence and nocturnal defecation.

Abdominal pain, nausea and vomiting, bloating, tenesmus, rectal bleeding help localize site.

Note any relationship to diet, fever, loss of weight or appetite, arthritis, or recent drugs. Small volume diarrhea with increased frequency, urgency and tenesmus suggests rectosigmoid disease. Large volume diarrhea suggests secretory component and usually involves small bowel with or without colonic involvement.

Acute diarrhea is usually infectious and self-limited. No work-up is needed.

Usual causes are infectious pathogens or inflammatory bowel disease. Lactose intolerance and drug-induced diarrhea are common. Many liquid medications are mixed in sorbitol, which is a laxative. Diabetic diarrhea is seen in longstanding diabetes.

Paradoxical diarrhea secondary to fecal impaction occurs in elderly or mentally ill patients. Thus all diarrhea in such patients needs a rectal exam and KUB.

Work-up: chronic and recurrent diarrhea should always be investigated, especially in cases of bleeding, dehydration, or weight loss, or in the immuno-compromised patient. Check stool for WBC, fecal fat stain, o+p; do c+s, including for *Yersinia enterocolitica*; check for *Clostridium difficile* toxin. Request for E. coli O157:H7 in bloody diarrhea. Check stool electrolytes and osmolarity. Next is flexible sigmoidoscopy or colonoscopy; do EGD in selected cases. Perform hydrogen breath test to exclude lactose intolerance, then D-xylose test and small bowel biopsy. If extensive work-up is negative, check serum gastrin (gastrinoma), calcitonin, VIP (VIPoma), and urinary hydroxyindole acetic acid (carcinoid syndrome).

Treatment is based on etiology.

C. difficile diarrhea: discontinue antibiotics, and treat with metronidazole (250–500 mg po tid) or vancomycin (125–250 mg po qid) for 10–14 days.

Giardiasis: metronidazole 250 mg po tid x 7 d or quinacrine 100 mg po tid x 7 d.

Lactase deficiency: lactose-free diet or exogenous lactase.

Ileal disease or resection: cholestyramine 1 packet bid-qid.

Pancreatic insufficiency: low-fat diet and pancreatic enzyme supplements.
Inflammatory bowel disease: sulfasalazine, steroids and azathioprine.

GASTROINTESTINAL INFECTIONS

AMEBIASIS: Intestinal and hepatic disease respond to medical treatment. Give metronidazole 750 mg tid x 10–14 d followed by iodoquinol 650 mg po tid x 20 d *or* diloxanide furoate 500 mg tid x10 d.

TOXOPLASMOSIS: antibiotic treatment for severe cases, immunocompromised or pregnant patients. Give pyrimethamine x 4 weeks plus sulfadiazine x 4–6 weeks plus leucovorin to diminish toxicity.

ASCARIASIS: give mebendazole 500 mg single dose or piperazine citrate 75mg/kg x 2 d to a max of 4 g in adults and 2 g in children <20 kg.

TOXOCARIASIS: occurs especially in children. Treatment is supportive. Give diethylcarbamazine 3 mg/kg tid x 21 d *or* thiabendazole 50 mg/kg/d x 5 d to kill larvae. Steroids if pulmonary, ocular, cardiac or CNS involvement.

STRONGYLOIDIASIS: symptomatic infection in immunocompromised host.
Up to 86% mortality in disseminated disease. Give albendazole 400 mg/d x 3 d.

TRICHINOSIS: found in myocardium, CSF, brain, liver. Muscle biopsy may be needed for diagnosis. Steroids used for allergic reactions. Give mebendazole 200 mg/d x 5 d.

SCHISTOSOMIASIS: liver, lung, bladder, CNS involvement depending on species. Fever, chills, headache, hepatomegaly and eosinophilia may be present. If untreated, will progress to chronic stage, including liver cirrhosis and portal hypertension. Praziquantel 40–60 mg/kg x 1 d in divided doses is treatment of choice.
Corticosteroids may be needed for allergic reaction.

ECHINOCOCCOSIS: occurs via ingestion of food contaminated by dog feces.
Fever, hepatomegaly and eosinophilia. Hepatic cysts may become infected or rupture. ELISA and indirect hemagglutination assay. Casoni test not recommended. Treatment is mostly surgical.

HEPATIC CANDIDIASIS: mostly leukemic patients. Multicentric abscesses on CT. Responds to amphotericin IV in 60% of cases.

SMALL BOWEL BACTERIAL OVERGROWTH:
1. Augmentin 875 mg bid x 7–10 d; avoid ampicillin, neomycin, aminoglycosides.
2. Alternate cephalexin (keflex) 250 mg qid *plus* metronidazole 250 mg tid x 7–10 d.
3. Tetracycline 250 mg qid x 7–10 d may not result in response in 60% of cases.

WHIPPLE'S DISEASE: caused by *Tropheryma whippelli*. No consensus on treatment. Trimethoprim/sulfamethoxazole (160/800) for 6–12 months. Do intestinal biopsy to document eradication before stopping antibiotics.

TRAVELLER'S DIARRHEA: ciprofloxacin 500 mg po bid x 3 d.

GIARDIA DUODENALIS: symptomatic patients have diarrhea, abdominal pain, nausea, vomiting, and weight loss. CBC and electrolytes are usually normal unless accompanied by malabsorption. Diagnosis by duodenal aspiration; stool tests may yield false negative results. Metronidazole 250 mg tid x 7 d, or quinacrine 100 mg tid x 7 d. Immunodeficient patients may need metronidazole for 6 weeks to 6 months.

CHOLERA: Tetracycline 40 mg/kg/d (in 4 doses, max 4 g/d) x 2 d.

ISOSPORA BELLI: Trimethoprim/sulfamethoxazole 160/800 qid x 10 d, then bid x 3 wks.

CRYPTOSPORIDIUM: Mild, self-limited except in immunocompromised patients. Treatment is unsatisfactory: paromomycin 500 mg qid x 2 weeks.

BALANTIDIUM COLI: Human infection is rare but can be fatal. May be asymptomatic or cause appendicitis, diarrhea or rectal bleeding. Treatment: tetracycline 500 mg qid x 10 d, or metronidazole 750 mg tid x 7 d.
Also treat asymptomatic carriers to prevent spread.

BLASTOCYSTIS HOMINIS: Debatable if it causes symptoms. If choosing to treat, use metronidazole 250–750 mg po qid x 1 wk.

CONSTIPATION

Definition: Constipation means different things to different people including lack of urge, hard stools or infrequent, difficult and painful defecation. Less than 3 stools per week is considered constipation.

Common Causes: low-fiber diet, sedentary lifestyle, inadequate fluid intake, aging, gynecologic or pelvic surgery, anorectal dysmotility, DM, neurologic disorders, hypothyroidism, depression, irritable bowel syndrome, medications (calcium channel blockers, aluminum and calcium antacids, antidepressants, opiates, anticholinergics), and colonic tumors.

Diagnostic Work-up: stool for occult blood, CBC, routine chemistries, thyroid function tests, flexible sigmoidoscopy, air-contrast barium enema or colonoscopy and radiopaque marker transit. Defecography and anorectal manometry in selected cases.

Investigate bleeding and change in bowel habit for malignancy.

Acute constipation may signify bowel obstruction, which manifests as nausea, vomiting, distended abdomen, and multiple air-fluid levels on abdominal X-ray.

Treatment:

- Discontinue offending drugs.
- Treat hypothyroidism, diabetes and metabolic abnormalities if present.
- Increase fiber: may get bloating or excess gas with fiber, and benefits are limited. Start with eating whole wheat bread, bran cereals or raw bran (bran 6–20 g/d). Wheat husk (3 sachets each of 3.5 g/d) is close to natural fiber and is 80% fiber. May use commercial products like psyllium (Metamucil 1–2 tbsf bid), calcium polycarbophil (Fibercon 1–2 tab tid), or methylcellulose (Citrucel 1 tbsf qd to tid). Fiber is not indicated in megacolon, dementia or neurogenic constipation.
- Drink plenty of fluid (6–8 glasses/d).
- Bowel retraining.
- Prokinetic agents (cisapride 10–20 mg qid) should not be used in routine constipation.

- Judicious laxative use.

Lactulose (15 ml bid-tid) or sorbitol (10–20 ml tid) and reduce as needed.
PEG solution (GoLytely) 1–2 L/daily to weekly.
Milk of Magnesia (magnesium hydroxide): 30–60 ml; use lower doses for concentrated formulations, intermittently for mild cases. Magnesium sulfate is cheap but has a narrow therapeutic window.
Anthranoid laxatives (Senna) form soft stools and are harmless if used in single dose for relief of mild, temporary constipation.
Phenolphthalein is best avoided.

Docusate sodium (50–500 mg/d with water in divided doses) softens stools by stimulating fluid secretion in small and large intestine, but its efficacy is not established.

Fleet enema *or* glycerin suppository, or bisacodyl 10 mg suppository intra-rectal prn.

ABNORMAL LIVER ENZYMES

Predominant elevation of serum SGOT/SGPT indicates hepatocellular process. Predominant increase of alkaline phosphatase suggests extrahepatic obstruction or intrahepatic cholestasis.

History: EtOH abuse, IV drug use, tattooing, exposure to chemicals/toxins, sexual orientation, pruritus, fever, stool and urine color, and family history of liver disease.

Physical exam: body weight, stigmata of chronic liver disease, hepatosplenomegaly, ascites and edema.

Work-up: hepatitis profile, iron, copper and ceruloplasmin studies, serum ANA, anti-mitochondrial antibody (AMA), anti-smooth muscle antibody (anti-SMA), and alpha-fetoprotein. Ultrasound is better for extrahepatic obstruction. CT is superior for hepatic or pancreatic lesions.

Asymptomatic increase in liver enzymes in obesity usually indicates fatty liver.

SGOT is greater than SGPT in alcoholic liver disease. Both are < 500 IU/L.

Transaminases >500 IU/L suggest acute viral or ischemic hepatitis, drug-induced injury (e.g. acetaminophen) or autoimmune hepatitis. Alcoholics have a lower threshold for acetaminophen-induced liver toxicity.

High alkaline phosphatase in healthy females suggests primary biliary cirrhosis.

Low serum albumin/protein, cholesterol or high PT/INR suggests acute or chronic liver dysfunction. Normal liver enzymes and liver function tests may be seen in patients with cirrhosis.

JAUNDICE

H&P provides clues to etiology in most cases.

Overproduction of bilirubin: hemolysis, large hematoma.

Defective glucuronyl transferase: Gilbert's syndrome, physiologic jaundice of newborn, breast milk jaundice.

Hereditary defects of bilirubin excretion: Dubin-Johnson Syndrome and Rotor's Syndrome.

Intrahepatic cholestasis: hepatitis, cirrhosis, primary biliary cirrhosis, cholestasis of pregnancy, sepsis and TPN, postoperative, AIDS.

Extrahepatic cholestasis: bile duct stones/stricture, biliary/pancreatic cancer, pancreatitis, hemobilia.

Ask about onset and duration of jaundice including previous episodes, color of urine and stools, associated abdominal pain, nausea, vomiting, anorexia, weight loss, transfusions, IV drug use, tattoos, sexual orientation and number of sexual partners, medications in preceding weeks/months and exposure to industrial or farm chemicals. Abdominal pain suggests pancreatitis. Pruritus occurs in chronic biliary obstruction.

Past medical history of gallstones or inflammatory bowel disease. Any jaundice among family and friends at the same time. Family history of cirrhosis (Wilson's disease, hemochromatosis, alpha-1-antitrypsin deficiency).

Physical exam: threshold for clinical detection of bilirubin is 2 mg/dl. Look for cachexia, xanthomas (chronic cholestatic liver disease), hepatosplenomegaly, abdominal mass, tenderness, ascites, evidence of easy bruisability/bleeding, stigmata of chronic liver disease (palmar erythema, spider angiomata, Dupuytren's contractures, gynecomastia, testicular atrophy), and mental status changes. Courvoisier's sign (palpable, nontender gallbladder in patient with jaundice) is positive in cholangiocarcinoma.

Kayser-Fleischer rings are seen in Wilson's disease. Absence of the ring does not exclude Wilson's disease.

Work-up: Routine chemistries, liver enzymes, serum albumin, protein, bilirubin, cholesterol, PT, hepatitis A, B and C profile, serum iron, TIBC, ferritin, ANA, anti-SMA, serum copper and ceruloplasmin, 24-hour urinary copper excretion, serum alpha-1-antitrypsin and alpha-fetoprotein, RUQ ultrasound and/or CT. Further work-up includes liver biopsy and/or

ERCP. Order abdominal CT for suspected tumor. Need ERCP for checking biliary tree. If ERCP unsuccessful or unavailable, order percutaneous transhepatic cholangiography (PTC).

Young patients are likely to have hepatocellular disease, whereas elderly are more likely to have stones or malignancy.

Unconjugated hyperbilirubinemia in adults with no other abnormal liver tests suggests Gilbert's disease. In neonates, most common cause is physiologic neonatal jaundice.

Hemolysis with normal liver rarely causes bilirubin to go above 5 mg/dl. Total bilirubin above 5 mg/dl is usually predominantly conjugated. Bilirubin rarely exceeds 25 mg/dl in extrahepatic biliary obstruction.

Associated enzyme abnormalities provide clues to etiology. Predominant elevation of SGOT/SGPT suggests hepatocellular disease of viral, toxic, autoimmune, drug, alcohol, or metabolic origin.

Predominant increase of alkaline phosphatase suggests cholestatic etiology like drugs, obstruction, sepsis, primary biliary cirrhosis and primary sclerosing cholangitis (PSC). Check RUQ ultrasound including common bile duct (CBD) diameter. Normal CBD is <7 mm (intact gallbladder) but the normal is higher in post-cholecystectomy patients.

If direct hyperbilirubinemia, assess if intrahepatic or extrahepatic. Fever and leukocytosis suggest cholangitis due to extrahepatic obstruction. Asterixis and mental status changes suggest hepatic encephalopathy. Abnormal LFTs (high PT, low albumin and cholesterol) and ascites can occur in acute hepatitis and do not necessarily indicate end-stage chronic liver disease.

ASCITES AND SPONTANEOUS BACTERIAL PERITONITIS

Most common cause is liver cirrhosis. Differential diagnosis: CHF, neoplasms, nephrotic syndrome and tuberculosis. 15–20% of cases have non-hepatic etiology. Sudden ascites with abdominal pain suggests hepatic vein thrombosis.

Work-up: paracentesis (elevated PT not a contraindication); prophylactic FFP and platelet transfusion not indicated.

Ascitic fluid should be sent for cell count, Gram's stain, culture and sensitivity, albumin (first tap) and protein. Fluid amylase, LDH, cytology, triglycerides, AFB smear and cultures in selected cases. Inoculate blood culture bottles at bedside with 10 ml of fluid for bacterial cultures.

SAAG (Serum to ascites albumin gradient) >1.1 g/dl is seen in liver cirrhosis, alcoholic hepatitis, CHF, liver failure, Budd-Chiari syndrome, portal vein thrombosis, veno-occlusive disease and myxedema.
SAAG <1.0 g/dl makes portal hypertension unlikely and is seen in peritoneal TB or carcinomatosis, pancreatic ascites, bowel obstruction/infarction, nephrotic syndrome and lymphatic leak.
Fluid protein <1.0 g/dl suggests high risk for development of spontaneous bacterial peritonitis (SBP).

Treatment of ascites: Diuretics, sodium restriction (1–2 g/d) and EtOH abstinence. Fluid restriction is not necessary unless serum sodium falls below 125 mEq/L. Spironolactone (100–400 mg/d) is diuretic of choice. Start with spironolactone 100 mg po qd plus furosemide 40 mg po qd. If ineffective, gradually use additional diuretic dose (spironolactone 100+ furosemide 40 mg each step to a maximum of 400 mg and 160 mg, respectively), keeping the ratio between spironolactone and furosemide (100:40). Goal of diuresis is weight loss of about 2 lb/day. Monitor BP, mental status, serum electrolytes, BUN and creatinine. Stop diuretics and re-evaluate if patient develops encephalopathy, serum sodium <120 mEq/L, or serum creatinine >2 mg/dl.

Avoid IV diuretics (reduce GFR) and NSAIDs. Some patients develop mild renal tubular acidosis, but there are no data to support use of sodium bicarbonate. Avoid urinary bladder catheters just for accurate measurement of urine output.

Dietary noncompliance is a major cause of lack of response to diuretics. Check 24-hour urinary sodium. Patients excreting >88 mmol/d of sodium in urine should be losing weight if they are ingesting less than 2 g/d of sodium.

Ten percent of cases are refractory to medical treatment and may require intermittent therapeutic paracentesis. Large volume tap may be performed in large ascites or if medical treatment is ineffective. Albumin 25–50 g IV infusion (very expensive) for paracentesis more than 5L.

Dopamine infusion should not be used in refractory ascites.

Cell count > 500/mm^3 or neutrophil count > 250/mm^3 or culture positive indicate spontaneous bacterial peritonitis (SBP). Cell count > 10,000/mm^3 indicates secondary peritonitis.

Traumatic ascitic tap: Subtract 1 neutrophil for every 250 RBC to arrive at correct number.

Treatment of SBP: Cefotaxime 2 g IV q8 h x 7 d. Tap may be repeated at 48–72 hours if no clinical improvement. A decline of cell count by at least 50% implies response to treatment. Prophylaxis using norfloxacin (400 mg/d) may be used for patients at high risk for SBP.

OCCULT GASTROINTESTINAL BLEEDING AND IRON DEFICIENCY ANEMIA

Occult heme-positive stools seen in 1–3% of healthy adults >40 yrs. Only 20–40% of patients with significant colorectal adenoma (>1 cm) have heme-positive stools.

Acid-peptic disease of upper gastrointestinal tract is most common cause of occult bleeding, followed by gastrointestinal tumors. AVM, NSAID, and EtOH intake are common.

Occult bleed secondary to varices and diverticulosis is very rare.

Microcytic hypochromic anemia is a late stage of iron deficiency. Iron deficiency anemia may be present without evidence of overt blood loss.

Do colonoscopy on patients with heme-positive stools and/or iron deficiency. Diverticulosis causes massive but not occult bleed. Thirty to 35% of occult heme-positive subjects have adenomatous polyps; 8–12% have colorectal cancer. Polyps <1 cm are unlikely source of bleeding.

If colonoscopy does not explain occult GI bleed and/or iron deficiency anemia, do EGD. As many as 75% of patients with a "positive" colonoscopy may have another lesion on EGD. Hiatal hernia is a frequently overlooked cause for slow, chronic bleed. If no lesion on EGD, do small bowel biopsy during EGD to exclude malabsorption as cause of unexplained anemia. As many as 25% of celiac sprue cases present for first time in elderly, and iron deficiency anemia may be the sole clue. If all are negative, do small bowel barium series.

If work-up is normal for patients with iron deficiency anemia, give trial of oral iron supplementation. If no improvement, consider further work-up for malabsorption syndrome. If Hgb improves, consider small bowel enteroscopy or enteroclysis, abdominal CT, and intraoperative endoscopy.

PARALYTIC ILEUS

Usually seen postoperatively or in presence of electrolyte disturbances, drugs (narcotics, tricyclic antidepressants, antipsychotics, calcium channel blockers), intra-abdominal inflammation/infection (pancreatitis, appendicitis, abscess, perforated viscous), ischemic bowel, or systemic sepsis.

C/o nausea, vomiting, abdominal distention, and lack of flatus or bowel movement. Bowel sounds are feeble or absent. Plain X-ray of abdomen shows air throughout GI tract. Must distinguish from bowel obstruction. Bowel sounds may be high-pitched in obstruction and X-ray shows a paucity of bowel gas distal to site of obstruction. If unable to exclude by clinical and X-ray criteria, perform small bowel barium study to exclude obstruction. Passage of oral contrast into colon during abdominal CT suggests ileus.

Treatment includes treatment of the cause and NPO, NG suction, IV fluids, and maintaining fluid and electrolyte balance. Neostigmine (2 mg IV over 60 minutes), erythromycin (250–500 mg IV q 8 h) or cisapride (10–20 mg qid) may be used in post-op cases that do not respond to conservative treatment. Avoid neostigmine in patients on beta-blockers, with bradycardia or recent myocardial infarction. Monitor EKG during neostigmine infusion in other cardiac patients. Do not use erythromycin and cisapride simultaneously.

GASTROINTESTINAL DISEASES
Diseases of the Esophagus

DYSPHAGIA

Difficulty in swallowing (dysphagia) may be due to motor disorder or obstruction caused by peptic stricture, Schatzki's ring, Zenker's diverticulum or neoplasm.

Transfer or oropharyngeal dysphagia implies problem in transferring food bolus from oropharynx into esophagus. This occurs in CVA, neuromuscular problems of tongue and pharynx, and head and neck tumors. Patients may ignore symptoms for months or years.

Odynophagia is painful swallowing. Usually infectious, caustic (pills or lye) or traumatic in origin.

Globus hystericus is a constant sensation of a lump in the throat without evidence of organic pathology. Occurs in patients with anxiety.

History should include solid vs. liquid dysphagia (intermittent or progressive), and any accompanying pain, weight loss or bleeding. Solid dysphagia, especially for meat and bread, suggests obstruction. The patient may have to wash down food with water. Food may get impacted in esophagus.

Progressive dysphagia suggests stricture or esophageal cancer. Schatzki's ring is characterized by intermittent dysphagia. Dysphagia primarily for liquids suggests transfer dysphagia. Combined solid and liquid dysphagia suggests esophageal motility disorder, e.g. achalasia. Weight loss suggests achalasia or malignant etiology.

Work-up: start with esophagram with a barium pill for suspected esophageal dysphagia. Do rapid-sequence films or videotaping when transfer dysphagia is suspected. EGD is performed as initial test for odynophagia, bleeding or weight loss. Motor disorders are diagnosed by manometry.

Treatment of benign strictures and Schatzki's ring:
esophageal dilatation.
Treatment of achalasia: pneumatic dilatation and myotomy (endoscopic or surgical). Endoscopic injection of botulinum toxin provides short-term relief of achalasia, and is used in elderly or sick patients who may be unable to withstand surgery.
Treatment of transfer dysphagia: dietary manipulation and rehabilitation.

GASTROESOPHAGEAL REFLUX DISEASE

Gastroesophageal reflux disease (GERD), or heartburn, is not the result of excess acid, but acid in the wrong place. Approximately 44% of Americans have heartburn monthly, and 14% and 7% have heartburn weekly or daily, respectively.

GERD is caused by weak lower esophageal sphincter (LES), gastroparesis and weak esophageal peristalsis. Transient LES relaxation after meals is normal. Reflux is worsened by large fatty meals, smoking, lying in bed soon after meals and straining.

Typical symptoms: Heartburn and effortless regurgitation of acid into oropharynx. Atypical presentations include chest pain, hoarseness, asthma, sore throat, and chronic cough.

Physical exam is usually unremarkable in uncomplicated cases.

Diagnosis is based on clinical history. Usually no work-up is needed. Empiric trial of acid-suppressive therapy (double-dose PPI) is the quickest way to assess whether symptoms are GERD-related. EGD is indicated in longstanding GERD (>5 yrs) to exclude Barrett's esophagus, GERD refractory to conventional therapy, dysphagia and odynophagia, wt loss and GI bleed.

Twenty-four hour pH monitoring is helpful in determining if persistent symptoms are due to continued acid reflux despite adequate medical or surgical therapy. Esophageal manometry is used for pre-op evaluation prior to surgery.

Differential diagnosis: viral (herpes or CMV) or candida esophagitis in immunocompromised patients (AIDS, DM, corticosteroid therapy). More than one organism may be involved. Pill esophagitis frequently seen in young females taking tetracycline for acne, and in elderly subjects.

Complications: bleeding, stricture, Barrett's esophagus.
Barrett's esophagus is premalignant, and surveillance EGD every 1–2 yrs is recommended. Esophagectomy if high-grade dysplasia or cancer found on EGD.

Prevention: avoid going to bed for 2 hours after meals. Elevate head end of bed during sleep.

Quit smoking and avoid drinking EtOH and carbonated, caffeine-containing beverages.
Eat small meals, slowly. Avoid mints, chocolate, onions, tomatoes.
Avoid heavy lifting and straining. Treat any cough or constipation.

Treatment: acid suppression with histamine-2 receptor blocker or PPI (lansoprazole 30 mg q am, omeprazole 20 mg q am; higher doses needed in some cases). Unlike ulcers, continuous suppression is required and a single nighttime dose of histamine-2 receptor blocker may not be effective. Cisapride (Propulsid 20 mg bid to qid) is helpful. Both drug treatment and surgery are effective in maintaining remission.

Esophageal strictures can be dilated using dilators. Surgical treatment for GERD is effective. Nissen's fundoplication is the most common surgical procedure. It can now be done laprascopically.

DISEASES OF THE STOMACH

GASTRITIS

Gastritis is an inflammation of the gastric mucosa. There is a poor correlation between endoscopic and histologic findings.

H. pylori is associated with almost all cases of chronic antral gastritis B. It predisposes to the development of adenocarcinoma and lymphoma. The role of *H. pylori* gastritis in causing symptoms is controversial.

Stress gastritis occurs in severely ill patients. Prophylaxis with histamine-2 receptor antagonists (ranitidine 150 mg IV q 12 h or famotidine 20 mg IV q 12 h) or sucralfate (1 g po or per NG tube q 6 h) to prevent bleeding is indicated for patients with head trauma, mechanical ventilation, coagulopathy or extensive burns.

Drugs and radiotherapy may cause changes ranging from erythema to ulceration. NSAID gastritis can be healed by discontinuation of the drug. Patients on chronic NSAIDs require prophylaxis if they are elderly, have a history of peptic ulcer, upper GI bleeding or cardiac disease. Misoprostol (Cytotec 200 mcg bid to qid), proton pump inhibitors (omeprazole 20 mg po qd or lansoprazole 30 mg po qd) or high dose histamine-2 receptor blockers (ranitidine 300 mg po bid, famotidine 40 mg po bid) are effective for prophylaxis.

Alkaline reflux gastropathy is seen in patients with gastroenterostomy. Diversion of alkaline juice by surgery yields inconsistent results. The mucosal-protective drug, sucralfate (1 g po qid) may help symptoms.

Eosinophilic gastritis may be due to drug allergy, parasites or idiopathic. Emphysematous gastritis (gas in stomach wall) occurs due to bacterial infection of stomach. Gastric emphysema may be benign.

HELICOBACTER PYLORI

H. pylori colonizes the stomach of 10–80% of the population. It is associated with almost all cases of antral gastritis B and is the most common cause of peptic ulcers (80–95% of duodenal ulcers and 60% of gastric ulcers. *H. pylori* is also associated with increased risk of adenocarcinoma of the stomach and MALT-lymphoma. Its role in non-ulcer dyspepsia is controversial.

H. pylori is diagnosed by: 1) histopathology and/or urease testing of gastric biopsy; 2) *H. pylori* serology; 3) urea breath test; or 4) fecal antigen testing. Test for H. *pylori* in patients with present or past history of ulcers and MALT lymphoma.

Serology is useful for screening but not to document the eradication after anti-Helicobacter treatment. Young patients (<50 yrs) without bleeding or weight loss may be tested for *H. pylori*, and if positive, treat prior to further evaluation of dyspepsia.

Must test for presence of *H. pylori* before instituting treatment. Eradicate *H. pylori* in active or past peptic ulcer as well as MALT (mucosa-associated lymphoid tissue) lymphoma. Anti-Helicobacter treatment is not effective in documented non-ulcer dyspepsia. However, many experts recommend that *H. pylori* eradication treatment should be offered to all symptomatic patients who are positive for *H. pylori*.

Single antibiotic treatment achieves eradication of *H. pylori* in only 20% of cases. Therefore, multiple antibiotics are required. Metronidazole (M), clarithromycin (C), peptobismol (B), amoxicillin (A), tetracycline (T), and omeprazole (O) or lansoprazole (L) are used in various combinations.

Combination of M (250 mg qid), B (2 tab qid), and T (500 mg qid) x 2 wks is commonly used. Amoxicillin may be substituted for T, especially in children, to avoid staining of teeth, but it is less effective. The addition of high dose omeprazole or lansoprazole overcomes most resistance to this regimen. Side effects include nausea, taste problems, diarrhea, and candidiasis.

Dosepacks improve compliance.
PrevPac (lansoprazole 30 mg x 2 + clarithromycin 500 mg x 2 + amoxicillin 500 mg x 2 x 2) contains one day's therapy of a 14-d triple therapy bid regimen.

Helidac (bismuth subsalicylate 262.4 mg tabs 2 x 4 + metronidazole 250 mg x 4 + tetracycline 500 mg x 4) is a dosepack example of metronidazole-based 14-day regimen.

*Alternate regimens:
(M) 500 mg bid + (O) 20 mg bid + (C) 500 mg bid x 7 d.
Ranitidine bismuth citrate (Tritec) x 28 d + (C) 500 tid for first 14 days of treatment.
(O) 20 mg bid + (A) 1 g bid + (C) 500 mg bid x 14 d.
Post-treatment testing for *H. pylori* eradication may be done if no symptomatic response, severe or complicated PUD, or prior treatment failure.

PEPTIC ULCER DISEASE

Most ulcers are due to *H. pylori*. NSAIDs are close second. Gastrinoma (ZE syndrome) is responsible for a small fraction of ulcers.

Duodenal ulcer causes epigastric pain 2–3 hours after meals and around midnight. Patients "feed" their ulcers and become overweight. Gastric ulcer causes epigastric pain within 30 minutes of eating and the pain is increased by food. Patients have anorexia and weight loss. However, signs and symptoms of ulcer lack sensitivity and specificity.

History and physical alone cannot diagnose ulcers. Diagnosis can be achieved by upper GI series although endoscopy is the gold standard. Follow-up EGD after treatment is usually indicated for gastric but not duodenal ulcer to rule out malignancy.

Treatment of peptic ulcer is two-pronged:

    1. improvement of symptoms and healing of ulcer;

    2. prevention of recurrence.

Aluminum and magnesium containing antacids can heal ulcers.

Sucralfate (1 g qid or 2 g bid) heals ulcers without blocking acid secretion.

Single nighttime dose of histamine-2 receptor blocker is equally effective as divided doses: ranitidine or nizatidine 300 mg po qhs, or famotidine 40 mg po qhs.

Proton pump inhibitors (omeprazole 20 mg po q am or lansoprazole 30 mg po q am) accelerate healing of duodenal ulcer, but not much for gastric ulcer.

NSAID ulcers require standard treatment. If NSAID is continued, it delays healing with histamine-2 receptor blocker but not if PPI is used.

Prevention of recurrence: 1) eradicate *H. pylori*; 2) maintenance histamine-2 receptor blocker treatment if *H. pylori* negative ulcers, failure of *H. pylori* eradication, history of ulcer complications, frequent recurrences or giant ulcers. Use ranitidine 150 mg qhs, famotidine 20 mg qhs, cimetidine 400 mg qhs, or sucralfate 1 g bid; and 3) discontinue NSAIDs or start NSAID prophylaxis with misoprostol 200 mcg qid. PPI (lansoprazole 30 mg qd or omeprazole 20 mg qd) or double-dose histamine-2 receptor blocker treatment are also effective for NSAID prophylaxis.

Surgery is helpful in refractory ulcers or for complications like uncontrolled bleeding, refractory gastric outlet obstruction or perforation.

DYSPEPSIA

Dyspepsia refers to a constellation of symptoms including abdominal pain, bloating, fullness, nausea, vomiting, and early satiety. Ulcers are seen in 10–15% of these cases.

Empiric treatment is indicated in younger patients (<50 years) without alarm symptoms. Patients with reflux-like symptoms should get anti-gastroesophageal reflux disease treatment. Patients taking NSAIDs should discontinue the drug if possible and receive histamine-2 receptor blockers. Based on studies of safety and cost-effectiveness, the remainder should be tested for *H. pylori* infection using serology. If positive, start anti-Helicobacter treatment, as though peptic ulcer is present. If negative, start histamine-2 receptor blockers.

Patients without response to empiric treatment should undergo EGD.

Non-ulcer dyspepsia (NUD) is the presence of dyspeptic symptoms without any apparent cause despite appropriate investigations. The pathogenesis is poorly understood. *H. pylori* infection, dysmotility, gastroesophageal reflux disease, drugs, intestinal gas, heightened visceral sensitivity, and psychosocial factors are implicated.

It is a diagnosis of exclusion after a normal EGD or UGI X-ray, RUQ ultrasound and solid as well as liquid gastric emptying studies.

Discontinue drugs with potential for GI side effects. Antacids, sucralfate, pancreatic enzymes, antispasmodics, and anti-Helicobacter treatment don't help. Use intermittent courses of histamine-2 receptor blocker if patient benefits: ranitidine 150 mg bid; famotidine 20 mg bid; cimetidine 400 mg bid.

Cisapride (Propulsid 10–20 mg tid) can be effective. Tricyclic antidepressants lower pain threshold (imipramine 10–100 mg/d). Refer patient to a psychiatrist if obvious psychiatric problems are present.

DISEASES OF THE INTESTINE

MALABSORPTION SYNDROME

Includes maldigestion (defective nutrient digestion inside gut lumen) and malabsorption (abnormal absorption across the gut wall).

Luminal digestion is impaired in cases of deficiency of lipase (pancreatitis, Zollinger-Ellison syndrome), gastric surgery (defective pancreatic stimulation and mixing of food with pancreatic secretions), pernicious anemia, small bowel bacterial overgrowth, chronic liver disease (reduced bile salt synthesis and secretion), terminal ileum disease (impaired enterohepatic recirculation of bile salts).

Impaired absorption occurs due to intestinal mucosal disease (bowel resection, celiac sprue, tropical sprue, Crohn's disease, GI infections), brush border enzyme deficiency, lymphangiectasia, radiation enteritis and infiltrating tumors.

Patients present with abdominal pain, distension, watery diarrhea with greasy stools, weight loss, excessive flatulence, fatigue, anemia, and bone pains. Many patients may lack classic symptoms of diarrhea and weight loss.

Signs: muscle wasting; dry, pale skin with bruises/petechiae; thinning listless hair; koilonychia and smooth tongue (iron deficiency); hyperpigmented skin (Whipple's disease); blistering of skin (dermatitis herpetiformis associated with celiac sprue); peripheral edema (hypoproteinemia); bone tenderness (vitamin D deficiency).

Labs: CBC may show microcytic hypochromic anemia (iron deficiency), macrocytic anemia (B_{12} deficiency, folate deficiency, hepatic disease) or mixed anemia; low lymphocytes <1000/mm^3 (lymphangiectasia); or low CD4 count (AIDS). Peripheral smear shows hypersegmented neutrophils (B_{12} deficiency); Howell-Jolly bodies (celiac sprue and IBD), acanthocytic erythrocytes (abetalipoproteinemia).

Metabolic profile shows low serum albumin, protein, calcium and magnesium.

Do thyroid function tests (hyperthyroidism) and anti-gliadin antibody test (sprue).

Stools should be tested for ova and parasites and screened for fecal fat stain. If stool weight exceeds 200 g/d, further 72-hour stool for fats (normal <7 g/d, may go up to 14 g/d in diarrhea) should be done while patient is on at least 75–100 g/d fat diet.

D-xylose test is normal in maldigestion, but abnormally decreased in malabsorptive mucosal diseases. Schilling test is done to test for cause of B_{12} deficiency. Lactose hydrogen breath test is abnormal in lactose intolerance. Duodenal aspirate or lactulose hydrogen breath tests should be done in suspected small bowel bacterial overgrowth.

Imaging tests: abdominal X-ray (pancreatic calcifications) and small bowel series (diverticulosis, strictures, blind loop, Crohn's).

Small bowel biopsy is essential to diagnose mucosal disease.

Treatment includes nutritional repletion and treatment of the cause, e.g. gluten restriction (wheat, rye, barley and oats) in celiac sprue; antibiotics in Whipple's disease, small bowel bacterial overgrowth, tropical sprue and GI infections; aminosalicylates and immunosuppressives in Crohn's disease; acid suppression in Zollinger-Ellison syndrome. Cholestyramine is helpful in limited ileal disease but worsens diarrhea if ileal disease is extensive.

If the cause of malabsorption is untreatable or weight loss is severe, start high protein and low fat (50% reduction) diet. Medium chain triglycerides may be used as fat substitutes. Vitamin and mineral deficiencies should be corrected orally if possible, otherwise parenterally.

LACTOSE INTOLERANCE

Lactose intolerance does not necessarily mean lactose malabsorption. History and avoidance diets are poor predictors of lactose indigestion. Selective adult-type hypolactasia is the predominant cause.

The prevalence is 6–22% among Caucasians in the U.S., 50–80% among Hispanics, Ashkenazi Jews and African Americans, and 80–100% among Native Americans.

Patients tolerate yogurt well because lactose is digested by bacterial lactase. Daily ingestion of <240 ml of milk is tolerated by most adult patients with lactose indigestion. Patients may also adapt to lactose ingestion over time.

About 5% of adult patients claim that their symptoms are caused by milk products despite normal lactase activity in the small bowel.

Diagnosis is by hydrogen breath test. Lactose tolerance test may be used. Testing is done for patients with suspected lactose intolerance without response to lactose restriction, as well as for patients with irritable bowel syndrome, to exclude lactose intolerance as a cause of their symptoms.

Enzyme solutions or tablets containing lactase can be used to digest lactose-containing foods. In order to hydrolyze 90% of lactose contained in 1 liter of milk, 0.25 g Maxilact Lx 5000, 2 ml of Lactozyme 3000 L, 2.6 g of Lactaid, 0.64 g of Lactase A or 0.4 g of Lactase N are required.

Liquid Lactase: (Lactaid; 5–15 drops per qt of milk).
Lactaid tablets (1 to 3) should be chewed/swallowed with first bite of dairy food. Lactase capsules 250 mg (1 to 2 caps) taken with dairy product. SureLac and Dairy Ease chewable tablets (1 to 3) with milk product.

DISEASES OF THE LIVER

HEPATITIS A VIRUS

HAV causes acute but not chronic hepatitis. It is usually self-limited. Approximately 30% of cases are seen in children. Severity increases with age. Children rarely have jaundice, while most adults do.

HAV is spread through the feco-oral route via contaminated food, water or person-to-person contact. IV drug use has declined as a risk factor to less than 2% of cases. Transmission by blood is rare.

Infection starts with constitutional symptoms of malaise, anorexia, fever, nausea and vomiting. Jaundice may appear. Transaminases may exceed 1000 IU/L. Bilirubin and alkaline phosphatase may be elevated. Illness usually resolves in 3–4 weeks although abnormal enzymes may persist for several months. Fulminant hepatitis is rare.

Extrahepatic manifestations are rare (skin rash and arthralgias).
Atypical manifestations: 1) relapsing hepatitis without progression; 2) cholestatic hepatitis with jaundice and pruritus (responds to corticosteroids); 3) autoimmune hepatitis.

Treatment is supportive.

Active immunization is recommended for travelers 1 month before going to an endemic area, children and adults living in endemic areas, adults with high-risk behavior (e.g. homosexual partners, IV drug use), and patients with chronic liver disease. Two formalin-activated vaccines are available (Havrix and VAQTA). A booster should follow the initial dose at 6–18 months.

Passive immunoprophylaxis with immune serum immunoglobulin (ISIG) prevents infection in 90% of exposed subjects. It is recommended for a single trip to an endemic areas and household contacts of cases.

HEPATITIS B VIRUS

Risk factors: IV drug use, tattooing, homosexual sex partners, multiple transfusions, multiple sex partners and medical personnel.

May develop rash, arthritis, glomerulonephritis, polyarteritis nodosa.

HBV profile: IgM core antibody is present in acute phase while IgG is present in chronic hepatitis or past infection. HB_sAb indicates development of immunity. HB_eAg indicates ongoing viral replication and high infectivity.

PCR assay is available for HBV DNA in serum.

Co-infection with delta virus may occur. This defective virus requires the presence of HB_sAg for its replication.

Natural history: fulminant hepatitis occurs in 1% of cases. Acute infection goes on to chronic hepatitis in <5% of immunocompetent adults but >90% infants. Half of chronic carriers have active viral replication. About 15–20% of patients with active viral replication develop cirrhosis within 5 years.

Treatment: Primary goal is to prevent complications of chronic hepatitis B. Alpha-interferon 5 MIU s.c. qd x 4 months in patients with positive Hb_sAg, Hb_eAg, and HBV viral DNA, elevated serum ALT and chronic hepatitis on liver biopsy. Monitor liver enzymes monthly. Check HBV DNA and Hb_eAg at beginning and end of treatment and six months later. A "flare up" of increased enzymes may occur initially, but do not change dose unless jaundice or worsening of liver function. Remission is sustained in 25–40% cases. Lamivudine (Epivir-HBV) 100 mg po qd x 1 year is also effective.

Monitor chronic HBV patients with alpha-fetoprotein every 6 months and annual RUQ ultrasound for development of hepatocellular carcinoma.

Passive immunoprophylaxis is used immediately after needle stick or sexual exposure along with active immunization. Passive immunoprophylaxis also used after liver transplantation in HB_sAg+ patients.

HBV immunoglobulin (HBIG) should be given to newborns of Hb_sAg positive mothers at birth followed by recombinant HBV vaccine within 7 days and then at 1 and 6 months.

HBV vaccine has 95% efficacy.

Three doses of active HBV recombinant vaccines (Engerix-B and Recombivax) at 0,1 and 6 months in high-risk groups, e.g., health care workers, IV drug users and infants of infected mothers.

HEPATITIS C VIRUS

Risk factors: IV drug use, multiple transfusions, medical personnel. Risk of transmission from pregnant woman to newborn is 3–6%. Sexual transmission is rare.

Fulminant hepatitis is rare. Up to 85% develop chronic disease. One-third go on to cirrhosis. In contrast to HBV, cirrhosis may be a prerequisite for development of hepatocellular carcinoma.
Extrahepatic manifestations include essential mixed cryoglobulinemia (1–2%), membranoproliferative glomerulonephritis, and Porphyria cutaneatarda (PCT).

Hepatitis C is diagnosed by presence of HCV antibody using ELISA test and confirmed by RIBA test. Order PCR assay for viral RNA to confirm presence in blood.

Treatment: Alpha-interferon (3 MIU three times per week for 12–18 months) for chronic HCV infection in patients with abnormal liver enzymes and moderate to severe inflammatory activity or fibrosis on liver biopsy. Treatment for patients with less severe disease or those with cirrhosis should be individualized. Check HCV RNA by PCR at 3 months. If still positive, unlikely to respond. Should not treat decompensated cirrhosis. Alfa-interferon (Intron A, Roferon-A) can be used for treatment of acute HCV infection.
Offer Interferon treatment to patients with stable HIV infection and good clinical status.
Interferon may increase risk of graft rejection in transplant patients.

Interferon alfacon-1 (Infergen) is a synthetic interferon. Dose 9 mcg s.c. 3 times per wk. If no response in 12 wks, increase dose to 15 mcg s.c. 3 times per wk.

Patients with HCV plus PCT should have hepatic iron depletion by phlebotomy before starting interferon treatment.
Contraindications to alfa-interferon treatment: thrombocytopenia (<100 K/mm³), leukopenia (<3000 cells/mm³), autoimmune disorders, alcohol dependence, severe depression. Some use reduced dose of interferon if platelet count between 50–100 K/mm³.

Side effects of interferon include initial flu-like reaction (fever, headache, malaise), fatigue, depression and bone marrow suppression. Check TSH at baseline and 3 months. Monitor CBC q wk x 4, then q 2 wks x 4, then monthly.

If liver enzymes are not normal by 3 months, stop treatment unless HCV viral RNA is undetectable. Only 10–20% patients treated with 12-month course of alfa-interferon have a sustained response. Ribavirin plus alfa-interferon (Rebetron) is effective in fresh patients and in those who do not respond as well as those who relapse after responding to interferon alone.

Monitor chronic HCV patients with alpha-fetoprotein every 6 months and annual RUQ ultrasound for development of hepatocellular carcinoma.

Patients with HCV should be vaccinated against HAV and HBV.

NONVIRAL LIVER DISEASE

ALCOHOLIC LIVER DISEASE

Liver disease occurs after a lifetime threshold of EtOH consumption has been reached (600 kg for men and 150–300 kg for women). For men, it means drinking 8 beers, 1 L wine or 1/2 pint whiskey qd x 20 yrs.
Less than half of those crossing threshold develop significant liver disease.

Corticosteroids are effective in severe alcoholic hepatitis: prednisolone 40 mg/d x 30 d followed by 4 wk taper.

GRANULOMATOUS LIVER DISEASE

Mostly sarcoidosis or tuberculosis. Tuberculosis has caseating granulomas while sarcoid is noncaseating. Differential diagnosis: bacterial, fungal and parasitic infections, drugs and primary biliary cirrhosis. Work up: chest X-ray; cultures for brucella, mycobacteria, fungi; VDRL, PPD and ANA; hepatitis profile; serology for Q fever, brucella.

AUTOIMMUNE HEPATITIS

Occurs more in women. Presents with fatigue, jaundice and hepatomegaly. Transaminases increased greater than 5 to 10-fold. Hypergammaglobulinemia with predominant IgG fraction. Serum ANA, anti-smooth muscle antibodies (anti-SMA) or antibodies to liver/kidney microsomes (anti-LKM1) are present. Viral, drug or EtOH-induced liver disease as well as Wilson's disease, hemochromatosis, alpha-1 antitrypsin deficiency, autoimmune cholangiopathy, nonalcoholic steatohepatitis must be excluded.

Treatment: prednisone 60 mg/d x 1 wk, 40 mg/d x 1 wk, 30 mg/d x 2 wk then 20 mg/d. Alternate regimen: prednisone and azathioprine (prednisone 30 mg/d x 1 wk, tapered to 10 mg/d over 4–5 wks along with azathioprine 50 mg/d po).
Patients who do not improve in 2 weeks have high early mortality and should be considered for liver transplantation.

PRIMARY BILIARY CIRRHOSIS

High alkaline phosphatase in a healthy middle-aged female. RUQ pain and itching are common. AMA positive in 90%. Serum IgM and cholesterol are increased. Ursodeoxycholic acid (13–15 mg/kg/d) improves symptoms and liver histology.

WILSON'S DISEASE

Low serum copper and ceruloplasmin and high urinary copper. Young patients present with hemolysis or hepatic manifestations. First presentation may be fulminant hepatitis. Older patients present with neurologic complications.

D-penicillamine is drug of choice; alternate is zinc.

PRIMARY SCLEROSING CHOLANGITIS

Seventy percent of cases associated with ulcerative colitis and 7% with Crohn's disease. In contrast, only 2.4–4% of ulcerative colitis patients develop primary sclerosing cholangitis. Diagnosis is by ERCP. Increased risk for cholangiocarcinoma.

Antihistamines may not help pruritus. Use cholestyramine 4 g po bid to qid or phenobarbital 30–60 mg po qhs or rifampin 300–600 mg po per day in divided doses.

COMPLICATIONS OF LIVER CIRRHOSIS

HEPATIC ENCEPHALOPATHY

Precipitated by GI bleed, infection, drugs and electrolyte abnormalities. Treatment: identify and remove cause; 60 g protein restriction in mild cases; vegetable proteins preferred; no protein in severe cases; lactulose 30 ml bid or tid to have 2–3 semisolid stools/d *or* lactulose retention enema 300 ml in 700 ml water bid or tid.

Neomycin 4 g/d in divided doses for reducing bowel bacterial load; risk for nephrotoxicity and ototoxicity. Metronidazole is alternate antibiotic.

GI BLEED

May be due to varices or portal hypertensive gastropathy. 40–50% of known variceal bleeders presenting for acute bleed may be bleeding from non-variceal cause.

PRURITUS

Treatment: Cholestyramine (4g bid to qid) prevents reabsorption of bile acids; maximum dose 16 g/d. Rifampin 300–600 mg/d in divided doses. Antihistamines and phenobarbital are useful but have sedative effects also. Naloxone (0.2 mcg/kg/min x 24 h).

Actigall (ursodeoxycholic acid): 13–15 mg/kg/d.

HEPATORENAL SYNDROME

Defined as functional renal failure without intrinsic renal disease in patients with liver cirrhosis. There is oliguria (<800 ml/d), and elevated serum creatinine. Urinary sodium is low (<10 mEq/L) despite diuretic treatment. Must exclude renal obstruction, nephrotoxic drugs, infection, and hypovolemia due to diuretics or bleeding. Work-up includes urine analysis, bolus normal saline infusion (1.5 L) and renal ultrasound. Consider post-void residual bladder volumes in cases of suspected bladder obstruction.

Dialysis is not done except as a bridge to liver transplantation.

BONE DISEASE

Treatment: Vitamin D and calcium supplements.

SPONTANEOUS BACTERIAL PERITONITIS

May present only with altered mental status. For diagnosis and treatment, see chapter on ascites. Norfloxacin 400 mg/d is used for prophylaxis in patients awaiting liver transplantation.

LIVER TRANSPLANTATION

Orthotopic liver transplantation (OLT) means that the diseased liver is removed and replaced with a healthy liver from a cadaver. In heterotopic transplantation, the healthy liver is placed at an ectopic site, e.g. when the patient is too sick for OLT. Indications for OLT may vary between various transplant centers.

OLT is indicated for end stage liver disease due to any cause, hepatorenal syndrome, recurrent SBP, albumin <2.5 g/dl, PT >5 sec above control, serum bilirubin > 5 mg/dl, intractable pruritus, severe osteopenia, recurrent biliary sepsis, intractable ascites, recurrent encephalopathy or recurrent variceal bleed.

OLT is indicated for cirrhosis due to HCV (irrespective of viremia). For HBV, OLT is performed in patients without viremia. It is also performed for fulminant hepatic failure due to viral or toxic hepatitis or Wilson's disease. Other indications include alcoholic liver disease, primary biliary cirrhosis, primary sclerosing cholangitis, hemochromatosis, and autoimmune hepatitis.

OLT is performed for hepatocellular carcinoma with single lesion <5 cm. Some transplant for up to 3 lesions for a maximum total of 5 cm involvement.

Contraindications: active infection, extrahepatic malignancy, AIDS, severe cardiopulmonary disease.

Relative contraindications: age >65 yrs, HIV+ without AIDS, alcohol and IV drug dependence, and psychosocial problems.

Pre-op work-up: establish etiology; liver biopsy; exclude psychosocial problems; pulmonary function tests and stress thallium or coronary angiography; upper and/or lower endoscopy in selected cases.

Timing: OLT is usually delayed until no alternative is available. At the same time, do not wait for the patient to become too sick. The prognosis of OLT in latter cases is poor. Consult a transplant center if the serum albumin is <3.0, PT >3 sec above control or if ascites or encephalopathy present.

DISEASES OF THE GALLBLADDER
CHOLELITHIASIS and CHOLECYSTITIS

Gallstones occur in 8–20% of the population. Most common are cholesterol gallstones (85%). Risk factors include female sex, obesity, multiparity, rapid weight loss, Native American ethnicity, and terminal ileal disease (e.g. Crohn's disease). Pigment stones are uncommon (15%).

Fifteen percent of gallstone patients also have choledocholithiasis. 95% of patients with choledocholithiasis have gallstones.

Gallstones remain asymptomatic in over 80% of cases. Complaints of gas, flatulence, bloating, non-ulcer dyspepsia are not caused by gallstone disease.

Biliary colic is the most common manifestation of gallstone disease. The word "biliary colic" is a misnomer since the pain is not colicky but steady and subsides in a few hours. Physical exam and laboratory studies are unremarkable. If the pain exceeds 6 hours, suspect acute cholecystitis. Elevated serum bilirubin, amylase and alkaline phosphatase suggest concomitant choledocholithiasis. Oral cholecystogram is rarely used these days and the test of choice is RUQ ultrasound.

Acute cholecystitis presents with prolonged RUQ pain radiating to shoulder, fever, RUQ tenderness, and leukocytosis. A worsening of pain with fever and chills and WBC >15000/mm^3 suggests gallbladder empyema and urgent surgical consultation is warranted.

Ultrasound is accurate for diagnosing cholelithiasis but not cholecystitis. Gallstones may be absent in 5% of cases of acute cholecystitis. Radionuclide HIDA scan is the test of choice for acute cholecystitis. Lack of filling of gallbladder with contrast indicates acute cholecystitis (95% accurate), while filling of gallbladder excludes it.

Admit patient with acute cholecystitis to hospital. NPO, IV fluids are started. NG tube suction if abdominal distension and vomiting. Consider antibiotics (cefoxitin in mild, whereas ampicillin plus aminoglycoside *or* third generation cephalosporin plus metronidazole in severe cases). Consult surgeon.

Treatment of acute and chronic cholecystitis is cholecystectomy.

Routine prophylactic cholecystectomy for incidental cholelithiasis is not recommended, even in diabetics. Exceptions include: 1) the risk of gallbladder cancer is high, e.g. calcified gallbladder, gallbladder polyp >1 cm in diameter, and young, Native American females; 2) young sickle cell patients; 3) patients awaiting organ transplantation; and 4) prolonged space travel or foreign travel to remote areas.

DISEASES OF THE PANCREAS

PANCREATITIS

Alcoholism and gallstones account for most cases. Differential diagnosis includes drugs (thiazides, sulfonamides, azathioprine, metronidazole, tetracycline, nitrofurantoin, valproate, corticosteroids, estrogens, furosemide, pentamidine), trauma, vasculitis, post-ERCP, hypercalcemia, hypertriglyceridemia, acute burns, long distance runners, HIV and other viral infections. Penetrating duodenal ulcer as a cause is very rare.

Ask about prior history of pancreatitis, alcohol use, and gallstones. Patients have epigastric pain radiating to the back with nausea, vomiting, low-grade fever, abdominal tenderness and distention.

Work-up: CBC, chem panel, serum lipase and amylase levels; abdominal X-ray series to exclude obstructed/perforated viscus; RUQ ultrasound for gallstones. Acute pancreatitis is a diagnosis of exclusion.

Differential diagnosis includes perforated viscus, ischemic bowel, leaking aortic aneurysm and renal colic. Serum amylase may be elevated in intestinal obstruction and perforation, mumps (salivary amylase), ectopic pregnancy, after ERCP or abdominal surgery. Serum lipase may be elevated in renal failure and acute abdominal conditions.

Initial management is supportive. Control pain with meperidine (50–100 mg IM q 3–4 h prn). Make patient NPO and maintain fluid and electrolyte balance. NG tube is needed only if patient is vomiting. Watch for signs of EtOH withdrawal and institute prophylaxis for delirium tremens (DTs) in alcoholic patients. Antibiotics and histamine-2 receptor antagonists are not routinely indicated.

Use Ranson's criteria to assess severity. Ranson's criteria at admission : 1) age >55 years; 2) WBC >16,000/mm^3; 3) glucose >200 mg/dl; 4) LDH >350 IU/L; and 5) AST >250 IU/L. Additional criteria during first 48 hours: 1) hematocrit decrease >10 mg/dl; 2) BUN increase >5 mg/dl; 3) calcium <8 mg/dl; 4) PaO$_2$ <60 mm Hg; 5) base deficit >4 mEq/L; and 6) fluid sequestration >6 L.

Admit patients with 3 or more Ranson's criteria to ICU and consult surgeon. Long acting narcotics, e.g. morphine or hydromorphone, are preferable to meperidine if large amount of narcotics needed.

Emergent ERCP for patients with impacted bile duct stone and cholangitis not responding to conservative treatment within 12–24 hours.

Early complications: hypotension, ARDS, renal failure, infection.

Start refeeding when pain and tenderness improves and patient is hungry. Start with small feedings of high carbohydrate diet. TPN for nutritional support if slow recovery. Include lipids in TPN unless triglyceride levels >500 mg/dl.

Get abdominal CT if infection is suspected or if patient does not improve. Follow-up serum amylase/lipase levels do not correlate with clinical status.

Elective cholecystectomy performed for gallstone pancreatitis after cooling off period during same hospitalization in most patients. Alcohol abstinence required for patients with EtOH pancreatitis. Consider surgical, endoscopic or radiological drainage of enlarging or symptomatic pseudocyst (>5 cm) if it persists for >6 weeks to prevent bleeding, rupture or infection.

Treatment of chronic pancreatitis: pain relief by analgesics, histamine-2 receptor blockers, discontinuation of EtOH, and pancreatic enzyme supplements (minimum 30,000 lipase units with each meal). Relieve any obstruction/stones in pancreatic duct. Surgical decompression of pancreatic duct or resection, and neural blocks may help.

DISEASES OF THE LARGE INTESTINES

DIVERTICULOSIS AND DIVERTICULITIS

Diverticulosis occurs mainly in the sigmoid colon and has been attributed to low-fiber diets. It is asymptomatic in 90% of patients. Usually detected on barium enema or sigmoidoscopy.

- Painful diverticular disease: crampy LLQ pain, constipation and tenderness. No fever or increase in WBC.
  Treatment: increase dietary fiber, dicyclomine (Bentyl) 20 mg po qid.

- 25% of patients with painful diverticular disease eventually get diverticulitis. Fever, tenderness in LLQ, leukocytosis with left shift. Pericolitis may affect adjacent organs (dysuria, frequency and urgency of urination).

Watch for peritoneal signs, order blood culture and sensitivity, check abdominal X-ray for free air. RLQ ultrasound and CT help to rule out abscess. Colonoscopy is contraindicated in acute, severe cases; it is performed after resolution to exclude concomitant malignancy (10% chance).

Treatment: patients with minimal symptoms are treated as outpatients with clear liquids and antibiotics (ciprofloxacin 500 mg po bid + metronidazole 250 mg qid for 7–10 d). Patients with significant symptoms or the elderly are hospitalized. Order NPO, IV fluids, and broad-spectrum antibiotics. Use ampicillin 500 mg IV q 6 h *or* cefoxitin 2 g IV q 8 h in mild cases. If severe, cefoxitin 2 g IV q 8 h + metronidazole 500 mg IV q 6 h + gentamicin 80 mg IV q 8 (adjust peak/trough). Symptoms usually abate in 3–4 d. Recurrence occurs in 20–30% after first episode and 50% after second episode.
Meperidine may be used for pain control if needed.

Consider surgery of acute cases if there is no resolution, or if there is worsening or frank perforation. Perform elective surgery in cases of young patients, recurrence (after second episode), fistula, or bowel obstruction.

- Diverticular bleeding is usually sudden, massive and usually from tics in right colon. Diverticulitis is usually not associated with bleeding. Occult bleeding is extremely rare.

IRRITABLE BOWEL SYNDROME

Most common GI condition referred to gastroenterologists.

Defined as abdominal pain for 3 months relieved with defecation or associated with change in consistency or frequency of stools. There may be bloating, mucus with stools, and change in stool form (lumpy, hard or watery), or defecation (straining, urgency or incomplete).

IBS less likely if old age, nocturnal symptoms, weight loss, fever, or bleeding.

Work-up patients to exclude other organic causes: CBC, ESR, hemoccult stools, stool for o+p and c+s, flexible sigmoidoscopy and lactose tolerance test. Colonoscopy, whole gut transit and imaging studies are done based on clinical situation.

Treatment: avoid carbonated beverages, chewing gum, caffeine, lactose, artificial sweeteners and any foods that worsen symptoms; high fiber diet with bran 2 tsp qid. May get increased symptoms due to gas. OTC fiber psyllium (Metamucil, Konsyl) or methylcellulose (Citrucil) may produce less gas.

Treatment of diarrhea: loperamide 1–2 tab tid, cholestyramine 1–4 packs qd. Lomotil in severe cases (up to 1–2 tabs qid and reduce asap).
Treatment of constipation: increase fiber and fluid intake; use stool softener.
Treatment of cramps: dicyclomine 10–20 mg po tid; hyoscyamine 0.125 mg po or sublingual.
Treatment of gas and bloating: simethicone or Beano (alpha galactosidase).

Severe cases benefit from low-dose antidepressants (e.g. amitriptyline or imipramine 10–100 mg/d) and psychotherapy.

COLON POLYPS AND CANCER

Be aware that different professional organizations have published guidelines that differ in recommendations for screening and surveillance of colon cancer.

Adenomas are premalignant. Hyperplastic polyps are inconsequential. Inflammatory polyps are seen in IBD. Juvenile polyps are seen in young patients and present as bleeding.

Risk of progression to cancer varies with pathology of adenomatous polyps (villous 40%, tubulovillous 22%, tubular adenoma 5%).

Annual fecal occult blood testing (FOBT) and screening flexible sigmoidoscopy is recommended >50 years in average-risk subjects. If sigmoidoscopy is normal, repeat in 5 years. If FOBT is positive or adenoma is present on sigmoidoscopy, perform colonoscopy.
If single, small adenoma (<1 cm) on colonoscopy, repeat colonoscopy at 3 years. If 3-year exam is negative, sigmoidoscopy every 5 years.
If large adenoma (>1 cm) or multiple adenomas on colonoscopy, repeat colonoscopy at 3 years. If 3-year exam is negative, repeat colonoscopy every 5 years.

Surveillance may be discontinued if it is unlikely to prolong life or life expectancy based on age and co-morbid factors.
Colonoscopy may be repeated 1 year after index colonoscopy if the initial exam was suboptimal or large or multiple adenomas were found.

If hyperplastic polyp is found on flexible sigmoidoscopy, no colonoscopy is required. The frequency of finding adenomas on colonoscopy is independent of the indication (e.g. heme-positive stools, family history of colon cancer) for colonoscopy.

Screening flexible sigmoidoscopy in asymptomatic patients above 40 years yields adenomas in 10–15%. Adenoma seen on sigmoidoscopy increases the possibility (30–50%) of proximal adenomas. Thus, a colonoscopy is indicated to examine the rest of colon. Frequency of colonic adenomas in asymptomatic subjects >50 years is 29%.

Perform colonoscopy at age 40 (or 10 years before the youngest case) in patients with family history of adenoma or colon cancer in a first degree relative <60 years, or two or more first degree relatives of any age. Repeat colonoscopy every 5 years.

Screening colonoscopy for high-risk subjects (e.g. inflammatory bowel disease), history colon cancer in first degree relative or familial adenomatous polyposis). In case of IBD, a colonoscopy every 1–2 years is recommended after 8 years of pancolitis, and 12–15 years of left-sided colitis.

Complete endoscopic excision of a polyp with severe dysplasia or carcinoma in situ is curative. Endoscopic excision of a polyp with invasive carcinoma is adequate in cases of well-differentiated or moderately-differentiated carcinoma with clear margins, and without involvement of submucosa or blood and lymphatic vessels. Surgical resection is recommended in cases of poorly differentiated carcinoma, extension into the submucosa or the blood or lymphatic vessels, and if polypectomy margin is involved (within 2 mm).

For patients with curative resection of colon cancer, perform colonoscopy if not done preoperatively. This is followed by colonoscopy or ACBE+flexible sigmoidoscopy at 1 year and 3 years. If normal, repeat every 5 years.

Please also see page 84 for colorectal cancer.

ISCHEMIC COLITIS

Risk factors: age >50 years, arrhythmias, hypotension, peripheral vascular disease, smoking, birth control pills and cocaine.

Most often watershed areas of splenic flexure or sigmoid colon.

There is abrupt onset of abdominal pain, rectal bleeding, and low-grade fever. Exam shows tenderness over the involved region of colon. Peritoneal signs are generally absent.

Admit patient to the hospital. Monitor vital signs and perform abdominal exam frequently. Follow abdominal X-rays. Perform flexible sigmoidoscopy to assess pathology. Angiography is of little value, but helpful if acute superior mesenteric arterial occlusion is also suspected.
Treatment is conservative: NPO, intravenous hydration and broad-spectrum antibiotics.

Start diet slowly. Advance as tolerated. Most patients recover spontaneously.
Surgery is indicated if bowel infarction or peritonitis.

Perform colonoscopy in 2 months to exclude cancer (10% chance) or residual stricture.

ANTIBIOTIC-INDUCED COLITIS

Occurs within a few weeks of antibiotic treatment. May occur with any antibiotic, especially clindamycin, ampicillin and cephalosporins. It may involve small intestine, colon, or both. May cause an asymptomatic carrier-state, mild diarrhea or severe pseudomembranous colitis (PMC).

Diagnosis is by history, *C. difficile* toxin assay and endoscopy. Approximately 3% of healthy adults are *C. difficile* toxin-positive carriers. PMC lesions on endoscopy are pathognomic. Flexible sigmoidoscopy is adequate in 2/3 of cases. However, 1/3 of cases occur only on the right side of the colon and may be missed by sigmoidoscopy.

Mild cases respond to discontinuation of the offending antibiotic. For severe cases, discontinue antibiotics, institute supportive care and metronidazole (250–500 mg po tid) *or* vancomycin (125–250 mg po qid) x 14 days; metronidazole 500 mg IV q 6 h may be used if oral drug is not tolerated. Do not use IV vancomycin.
Approximately 20% of responders have relapse but most respond to repeat course of same antibiotic. Rate of relapse is not influenced by choice of antibiotics.

If antibiotics have to be continued, use systemic antibiotics less likely to cause PMC (e.g. aminoglycosides, bactrim, erythromycin, or quinolones).

INTESTINAL ANGINA (ABDOMINAL ANGINA)

Rare cause of abdominal pain. Usually due to atherosclerosis. Recurrent abdominal pain occurs within 30 minutes after eating and is associated with fear of eating and weight loss. Abdomen is not tender even during the pain. Abdominal bruit may be heard.

Diagnosis is clinical and is supported by angiography plus response to revascularization. Exclude other causes of GI pain before vascular work-up. Mere stenosis of the splanchnic arteries does not establish diagnosis.

Treatment is surgical revascularization. Benefit occurs when at least two of the three major vessels (celiac, superior mesenteric and inferior mesenteric arteries) are involved on angiography.

ACUTE MEGACOLON AND OGILVIE'S SYNDROME

Acute megacolon occurs due to inflammatory, infectious or distal obstructive process (e.g. volvulus) in the colon. Ogilvie's syndrome is colonic pseudo-obstruction and occurs due to trauma, postoperative, electrolyte and neurologic problems.

Abdominal pain and distension are present. WBC counts are normal. Abdominal X-rays show massive dilatation of colon. Fever, peritoneal signs and leukocytosis are uncommon and require urgent surgical exploration.

Keep patient NPO and start IV fluids, NG tube suction, rectal tube and rectal enemas. Correct serum electrolytes, calcium and magnesium. Glycemic control is important in diabetics. Check thyroid function tests. Water-soluble contrast enema is diagnostic and may be therapeutic if obstruction is suspected. Most patients resolve with this treatment.

Neostigmine (2 mg IV over 60 min), erythromycin (250–500 mg IV q 8 h), metoclopramide (Reglan 10–20 mg IV q 8 h) or cisapride (Propulsid 20 mg po qid) dosing may be used in nonresponders after excluding bowel obstruction. Neostigmine is contraindicated in patients on beta-blockers, with bradycardia, or history of a recent MI. Monitor EKG during neostigmine infusion in other cardiac patients. Do not use erythromycin and cisapride simultaneously.

Conservative management for 24 hours, then colonoscopic decompression if cecal diameter exceeds 11 cm. Failures require surgical consultation.

CHRONIC INTESTINAL PSEUDO-OBSTRUCTION

Clinical syndrome caused by primary or secondary myopathies (sclero-derma, polymyositis, radiation), neuropathies (diabetes mellitus, paraneoplastic syndrome, Chagas' disease, Parkinsonism), small intestinal diverticulosis, endocrine disorders (hypothyroidism, hypoparathyroidism, pheochromocytoma), and drugs (opiates, antipsychotics and antidepressants).

Pseudo-obstruction involves more than one part of GI tract. Approximately 75% have esophageal involvement. There is variable presentation of abdominal pain, distension, nausea, vomiting, and constipation. Symptoms may be intermittent.

Work-up: Lab tests reflect malnutrition. Abdominal X-ray and barium studies of entire GI tract to exclude obstruction. Use manometry in selected cases, and exploratory laparotomy if obstruction can't be excluded.

Treat cause if possible; discontinue offending drugs.
Low residue, low fat, and low lactose diet.
Drug options: cisapride (Propulsid) 20 mg qid; octreotide 50 mcg qhs with or without erythromycin 200 mg po tid; antibiotics in stagnant loop syndrome.

Heller's myotomy, venting gastrostomy, feeding jejunostomy, or total abdominal colectomy with ileoanal anastomosis in selected cases.

MELANOSIS COLI

Occurs mainly in elderly subjects and is usually an incidental finding during sigmoidoscopy or colonoscopy. It is caused by chronic use of anthracene laxatives (cascara, senna) and herbal teas. Incidence is rising.

It is a benign, reversible condition of no proven clinical significance. However, it is a marker for the potential development of cathartic colon due to cathartic abuse and its presence carries a 3-fold increased risk of colon cancer.

There is no specific treatment. Reverses after offending laxative stopped.

INFLAMMATORY BOWEL DISEASE
(ULCERATIVE COLITIS, CROHN'S DISEASE)

Infections, drugs, C. *difficile* toxin, radiation and ischemia may cause inflammation in the bowel. Usually when we say IBD, we imply chronic idiopathic inflammation.

Although considered a disease of the young, there is a second peak at 70 years.
IBD comprises ulcerative colitis (UC) and Crohn's disease (CD). Type may be indeterminate in 10–15% cases.

Ulcerative colitis (UC) involves rectum in 95% of cases and advances proximally. The extent of proximal advancement is variable, e.g. it may be left-sided UC or pancolitis. UC in elderly is usually limited to rectosigmoid region and is rarely pancolitis.

Usual presentation of UC is bloody diarrhea, abdominal cramps and urgency.
Assess volume, blood and nutritional status. Abdominal tenderness in moderate to severe cases. Patients with severe colitis have tachycardia, anemia, hypoalbuminemia and >10% weight loss. Peritoneal signs (rebound, guarding, rigidity) suggest fulminant colitis. Diagnosis is by endoscopy. Crypt abscesses on histology.

Crohn's disease (CD) may involve any part of GI tract from mouth to anus and the disease may be patchy. Approximately one-third of cases each involve small bowel only, colon only, and both small and large bowel. Rectum is usually spared. CD in elderly usually involves colon only.

Patient may have predominantly inflammatory, obstructive or perianal Crohn's disease. Chronic inflammation leads to fibrosis and strictures. Fistulae may connect the bowel with another loop of bowel or bladder, vagina, or skin.
Presentation of CD varies with the site and degree of involvement. It may be gradual in onset with episodes of abdominal pain, diarrhea (may be bloody), low-grade fever.
Exam may show RLQ mass and tenderness, anal fissures, perianal abscess or fistulae.
Diagnosis of Crohn's disease is based on clinical picture, imaging studies and endoscopic findings. Small bowel X-ray may show inflammation, ul-

cers, strictures or fistulae. Colonoscopy shows inflammation with aphthous or linear ulcers, patchy inflammation, fistulae or strictures. Granulomas are seen on histology in half the cases. Order CT of abdomen to exclude an abscess if patient has tender abdominal mass with fever and leukocytosis.

Extra-GI manifestations of IBD include arthritis, uveitis, hepatitis, primary sclerosing cholangitis. Gallstones and renal stones occur in CD.

IBD has increased risk for colon cancer and the risk depends on extent and duration. Colonoscopy every 1–2 years is recommended after 8 years of pancolitis and 12–15 years of left-sided colitis.

Sulfasalazine is cornerstone of treatment. Dose 500 mg to 1 g po qid. There is dose-response relationship. Newer, less toxic 5-ASA compounds, mesalamine (Asacol 1.6 to 4.8 g/d po and Pentasa 4 g/d po) and olsalazine (Dipentum 0.75 to 1.5 g/d) are available. Use plenty of water with these drugs.

Steroids induce, but do not maintain, remission. Azathioprine or 6-MP (1–2.5 mg/kg/d po) is useful in steroid-dependent disease as well as perianal Crohn's disease. However, azathioprine/6-MP may take 3–12 months to have its effect. Loading dose of azathioprine (50 mg/h IV x 36 h), followed by regular oral dosing results in more rapid response within weeks. Monitor CBC while on azathioprine.

Cyclosporine is effective in toxic megacolon due to UC (4 mg/kg/d IV) as well as inflammatory/fistulous Crohn's disease (4 mg/kg/d IV or 5–7.5 mg/kg/d po). Cyclosporine has dose-dependent nephrotoxicity.

Metronidazole (500 mg po bid to qid) and ciprofloxacin (250 mg po tid), alone and combined, are useful in Crohn's disease, especially perianal fistulae. Watch for peripheral neuropathy due to metronidazole.

Infliximab (Remicade 5 mg/kg single IV infusion over 2 hours) is used for moderate to severe active Crohn's disease unresponsive to conventional treatment. The initial dose is repeated at 2 weeks and 6 weeks for fistulizing Crohn's disease.

Surgery is curative in ulcerative colitis. Incision and drainage of abscesses and resections are needed in Crohn's disease.

DISEASES OF THE ANUS AND RECTUM
ANORECTAL DISEASES

Complaints include perianal pain, itching, bleeding, and protruding mass.

HEMORRHOIDS and ANAL FISSURES

Internal hemorrhoids arise from superior hemorrhoidal vascular plexus above pectinate line and are covered with mucosa, whereas external hemorrhoids arise from inferior hemorrhoidal vascular plexus below pectinate line, and are covered with skin. Most patients have mixed disease and present with bleeding (usually on side of stool) or prolapsing mass. Itching is due to poor perianal hygiene and not hemorrhoids. Pain is not present unless sudden prolapse of internal hemorrhoid. Sudden, throbbing pain with tense bluish hemorrhoidal lumps suggest thrombosed external hemorrhoid. Chronic iron deficiency anemia may result from hemorrhoidal bleeding.

Inspection and digital rectal exam are essential for physical exam. Anoscopy for visualization of anal canal and flexible sigmoidoscopy should be performed in all patients with anorectal complaints.

Anal fissure is a tear in anal canal starting from anal verge and occurs mostly in women. It is usually in posterior midline position. Other locations suggest Crohn's disease or cancer.

Treatment of hemorrhoids and anal fissure:

> High fiber diet (Metamucil/Citrucel dosing) and plenty of water (8 glasses/d).
>
> Stool softeners; emollient suppositories and ointments.
>
> Sitz bath; avoid prolonged sitting on toilet.
>
> Topical nitroglycerine 0.5% for fissure.

Sclerosants and band ligation are used for hemorrhoids.
Surgery is indicated for Grade 4 hemorrhoids and recurrent fissures.
Treatment of thrombosed hemorrhoid:

> Excision performed in first 48 hours.
>
> If presentation after 48 hours, observe (symptoms aba′e).

SOLITARY RECTAL ULCER SYNDROME (SRUS)

SRUS may not be solitary, or limited to rectum. May not have frank ulceration.
Can have anal pain with blood and mucus per rectum.
Biopsy is diagnostic.
Treatment: bulking agents; avoid straining.

PRURITUS ANI

Etiologies include fecal leakage, anorectal disease, dermatologic disease, antibiotic diarrhea, fungal and parasitic (pinworm) infection, DM, liver cirrhosis, poor hygiene, foods (caffeine, alcohol, tomatoes, citrus, chocolate), psychogenic and idiopathic. Treatment is directed at the cause.

CHRONIC PERIANAL PAIN

Proctalgia fugax is sudden crescendo pain in upper anal canal, lasting a few minutes and worsened by anxiety. It occurs at night, usually in young males.

Coccygodynia is a constant aching sensation in perineum and anal canal of adult females, occurring during daytime. There may be tender spots in sacrococcygeal area.

Chronic idiopathic perineal pain is a dull, aching, throbbing or burning sensation in anal canal, intermittent or constant, worsened on sitting and relieved on lying down. It occurs in middle-aged to elderly females with prior history of pelvic or spinal surgery.

DISEASES IN SPECIAL PATIENT POPULATIONS

NSAIDS AND GI TRACT

Injury may occur throughout GI tract. Significant side effects in less than 4% per year.

NSAID gastropathy is more common than ulcers. Risk for ulcers is dose-related. Low-dose aspirin can cause serious complications.

Risk for serious GI complications is highest in first 6 months. If ulcer occurs, discontinue NSAID. If NSAID can't be discontinued, treat with high-dose histamine-2 receptor blocker (ranitidine 300 mg bid or pepcid 40 mg bid) or proton pump inhibitor (lansoprazole 30 mg qd or omeprazole 20 mg or bid).

Prophylaxis should be used for patients with history of peptic ulcer, upper GI bleed, concomitant steroid therapy, serious cardiac illness, and >70 years. Misoprostol is effective for NSAID prophylaxis against gastroduodenal complications; 200 mcg qid is more effective than 100 mcg qid but has more side effects. PPI and high-dose histamine-2-blockers are also effective.

Ibuprofen and diclofenac (Voltaren) are considered low-risk, while ketoprofen (Orudis) falls in high-risk category. Naproxen (Naprosyn), indomethacin and piroxicam (Feldene) fall in the intermediate category.

There is increased risk of perforation for patients with diverticulosis.

Chronic NSAID use reduces relative risk of colorectal cancer. Sulindac causes reduction of polyps in familial adenomatous polyposis.

Prevalence of sporadic adenomas in chronic NSAID users is lower. NSAIDs are not effective when used for secondary prevention of adenomas.

LIVER DISEASE IN PREGNANCY

Placental alkaline phosphatase is present, so normal serum value is doubled.

Viral hepatitis is the most common cause of jaundice.

Intrahepatic cholestasis of pregnancy

During third trimester: complaint of pruritus and jaundice.
Bilirubin < 5 mg/dl, high alkaline phosphatase, and normal or increased SGOT/SGPT.
Increased premature labor; recurs during future pregnancies.

Acute fatty liver of pregnancy (AFLP)

Occurs after 35th week of gestation.
Nausea and vomiting, headache, abdominal pain, bleeding, jaundice (coma).
SGOT/SGPT <750 IU/L; high bilirubin, alkaline phosphatase.
High WBC, serum creatinine and serum ammonia; low glucose; DIC may occur.
Supportive treatment; delivery lifesaving and done emergently.
Fetal and maternal mortality 20%.

HELLP syndrome

Occurs in 3rd trimester.
Hypertension, elevated liver enzymes and DIC.
Associated with preeclampsia.
Treatment: terminate pregnancy.

Viral hepatitis during pregnancy

Pregnancy has no effect on course of hepatitis.
More premature labor; more still births. High rate of transmission of hepatitis B virus to offspring, so immunization of newborn recommended (see chapter on hepatitis B virus).

AIDS PATIENT

Dysphagia and odynophagia are likely to be infectious. More than one organism may be present. Treat oral thrush with fluconazole 200 mg po loading and then 100 mg/d po. Fluconazole is more expensive but more effective than ketoconazole. If symptoms persist after 1 week, do EGD with biopsy and brushings.

Herpes simplex virus (HSV) esophagitis: acyclovir 250 mg/m^2 q 8 h x 7–10 d.
Use HSV prophylaxis with oral acyclovir if at risk for recurrence.
Cytomegalovirus (CMV) esophagitis: ganciclovir 5 mg/kg IV q 12 hr x 2 wks or foscarnet 60 mg/kg over 1 hr q 8 h x 2–4 wks.

Abdominal pain, nausea and vomiting, weight loss suggests CMV or obstruction by lymphoma.
EGD and small bowel series or enteroclysis if no response to histamine-2 receptor blocker.

Severe abdominal pain suggests pancreatitis or CMV-induced bowel perforation. HIV, AZT, ddi or Bactrim may cause pancreatitis.

Diarrhea affects many patients. Malabsorption syndrome may occur due to infections. Persistent infection may be caused by Cryptosporidia, Salmonella or *Campylobacter jejuni*. Stop medications that may cause diarrhea. Check stool for o+p, do c+s, and look for *C. difficile* toxin. If negative, do EGD with small bowel biopsy, flexible sigmoidoscopy or colonoscopy with biopsy and viral cultures.

Salmonella, Shigella, Campylobacter: ciprofloxacin 500 mg q 12 h x 10–14d.
Microsporidium: metronidazole 500 mg qid x 14 d.
Isospora belli: Trimethoprim/sulfamethoxazole 160/800 qid x 10 d, then bid x 3 weeks.

Treatment of unexplained diarrhea: loperamide or Lomotil or tincture of opium (0.6 ml po q 4–6h prn), cholestyramine, bulk-forming agents, and octreotide.

GASTROINTESTINAL CANCER

GI CANCER

ESOPHAGEAL CANCER
Clinical presentation: Progressive dysphagia with weight loss.
Diagnosis: Barium swallow shows irregular stricture. Endoscopic biopsy provides definitive diagnosis. Endoscopic ultrasound, chest and abdominal CT are used to look for metastases.
Histology: squamous cell carcinoma in proximal esophagus, and adenocarcinoma in distal end.
Treatment: radiotherapy, chemotherapy and curative resection in early disease.
Palliative treatments include resection, stent placement and laser treatment. Poor prognosis (5 yr survival <10%) even when no metastases seen.

GASTRIC CANCER
Type: 90% adenocarcinoma.
Outcome: Poor prognosis can be expected (5 year survival <10%) unless detected "early".

Diagnosis: Upper GI series shows an ulcer or a mass. Endoscopic biopsy provides diagnosis.

Work-up: chest and abdominal CT for metastases.

Treatment: curative resection in early stages.

SMALL BOWEL TUMORS
Relatively rare. Adenocarcinoma occurs more in proximal small bowel while lymphoma in distal small bowel. Carcinoid is a slow growing, locally metastatic tumor. It does not manifest as carcinoid syndrome unless hepatic metastasis is present.

Small bowel obstruction may be seen on abdominal X-ray, small bowel X-ray or enteroclysis. Diagnosis is by small bowel enteroscopy with biopsy or exploratory laparotomy.

Treatment is usually surgical. For lymphomas adjuvant chemotherapy is used.

COLON CANCER

Curative resection possible in early stages. After resection, perform colonoscopy or ACBE+Flex sig at 1 and 3 years. If normal, repeat every 5 years.

Adjuvant chemotherapy with 5-FU and levamisole is indicated for Duke's C colon cancer. For rectal cancer, adjuvant radiotherapy and chemotherapy for Duke's B2 and C is indicated. Camptosar (irinotecan) also improves survival in metastatic colorectal cancer. (See chapter on colon cancer for details)

GASTRINOMA or ZOLLINGER-ELLISON SYNDROME

Characterized by refractory, recurrent or multiple ulcers associated with increased gastric acid output, increased serum gastrin and non-beta islet cell tumor of the pancreas. About 0.1–1% of all duodenal ulcers are caused by ZES. Average delay between symptom onset and diagnosis is 6 years. Suspect it in patients with multiple or refractory or recurrent ulcers; non-*H. pylori*, non-NSAID ulcers; and in patients with ulcers and diarrhea or family history of ulcers.

Gastrinomas may be sporadic or associated with multiple endocrine neoplasia (MEN) type I . More than two-thirds of gastrinomas are malignant, 24% have hepatic metastasis at the time of diagnosis.

In patients with appropriate clinical picture, increased gastric acid output and fasting serum gastrin >1000 pg/ml is diagnostic. Secretin stimulation test is helpful in atypical cases.

Abdominal CT, endoscopic ultrasound, MRI and selective arteriography should be done to localize tumor.

Surgical resection is treatment of choice. Exploratory laparotomy with intent to treat is done even if tumor is not localized preoperatively, unless patient has unresectable hepatic metastasis. High-dose proton pump inhibitors (lansoprazole or omeprazole) are used during preoperative evaluation and if gastrinoma cannot be located or resected.

Family members of patients with MEN-I should undergo screening with serum fasting gastrin and secretin stimulation test.

PANCREATIC CANCER

Mostly adenocarcinoma and in head of pancreas.
Overall, prognosis is dismal (5 year survival 1%).

History: jaundice, pruritus, weight loss, dark urine, acholic stools.
Pancreatic mass and dilated bile ducts seen on ultrasound or CT; use ERCP if diagnosis is unclear. CT and endoscopic ultrasound used for staging and

vascular invasion. Whipple's procedure used for curative resection.
Palliation by biliary stents placed endoscopically or through PTC.

LIVER CANCER

Mostly metastatic tumors from GI tract, lung, breast and ovaries.
Primary cancer is hepatoma or hepatocellular carcinoma.
Risk factors are liver cirrhosis, HbsAg positive, HCV and hemochromatosis.

High alpha-fetoprotein occurs in hepatoma. Abdominal CT reveals tumor.
Multiple nodules suggest metastasis. Perform biopsy for diagnosis.

Hepatoma carries dismal prognosis.
Liver transplantation if lesion <5 cm.

Index

abdominal angina, 72
abdominal exam, 5
abdominal hemmorrhage, 26
abdominal MRI, 13
abdominal pain
  and acute megacolon, 73
  and determination of acuity, 3
  and diarrhea, 32
  and jaundice, 38
abdominal pain, acute, 26–28
abdominal X-ray, 12
achalasia, 12
  and dysphagia, 44
  and vomiting, 25
acid peptic disease, 42
acute cholecystitis, 13
acute dirrahea, 6
acute fatty liver of pregnancy (AFLP), 81
acute megacolon, 73
acute mesenteric ischemia, 10
acute pancreatitis, 12
acyclovir, 23
adenocarcinoma, 47
adenomas
  and colon polyps/cancer, 68
  and NSAIDs, 80
AIDS, 82
  and antibiotic prophylaxis, 18
  and common mistakes, 10
  and GERD, 45
  and jaundice, 38
  and liver transplants, 62
  and malabsorption syndrome, 52
air-fluid levels, 12
albumin, 7–8
alcohol
  and gastrointestinal bleeding, 30
  and hepatitis, 21, 57

and liver transplants, 62
and pancreatitis, 64
and pruritis ani, 79
See also EtOH
alkaline phosphatase
  and AFLP, 81
  and cholestasis, 7
  and HAV, 55
alkalosis, 19
alpha-1 antitrypsin deficiency, 38
alpha-fetoprotein
  and HBV, 56
  and liver cancer, 85
  and liver enzymes, 37
alpha-interferon
and HBV, 56
  and HCV, 57, 58
amebiasis, 33
aminosalicylates, 21
ampicillin, 71
anal fissures, 78
analgesia, 17
anemia
  and GI bleeding, 6
  and hemorrhoids, 78
  and iron deficiency, 42
  and malabsorption syndrome, 52
angiography, 13
  and abdominal pain, 27
  and acute mesenteric ischemia, 28
  and common mistakes, 10
  and intestinal angina, 72
  and ischemic colitis, 70
anorectal diseases, 78
anorexia
  and HAV, 55
  and jaundice, 38
  and peptic ulcers, 50
  and vomiting, 25

Title List from International Medical Publishing

ISBN — Title — Author — Price

Intern Pocket Survival Guides

0-9634063-0-2 The Intern Pocket Survival Guide–Masterson $7.50

0-9634063-1-0 The CCU Intern Pocket Survival Guide–Masterson/Rothenhaus $7.50

0-9634063-2-9 The ER Intern Pocket Survival Guide–Rothenhaus/Masterson $7.50

0-9634063-3-7 The ICU Intern Pocket Survival Guide–Masterson/Rothenhaus/Tenner $7.50

0-9634063-5-3 The Surgical Intern Pocket Survival Guide–Chamberlain $7.50

0-9634063-9-6 The Oncology Intern Pocket Survival Guide–Tenner/Masterson/Rollhauser $7.50

Emergency Handbooks

0-9634063-8-8 The EKG Pocket Survival Guide–International Medical Publishing $6.00

1-883205-16-6 The ACLS Pocket Survival Guide–International Medical Publishing $6.00

1-883205-19-0 The PALS Pocket Survival Guide–International Medical Publishing $6.00

1-883205-46-8 The Pocket Guide to Emergency and Disability Scores $6.00

1-883205-20-4 First Aid–Bureau of Mines $6.25

Clinical Practice Handbooks

1-883205-44-1 Pocketful of Prevention–Masterson $7.50

1-883205-39-5 The Gastroenterology Resident Pocket Survival Guide $9.95

Medical Student Titles

0-9634063-6-1 The Pocket Guide to Eponyms and Subtle Signs of Disease–Tenner/Masterson $7.50

0-9634063-4-5 The Intern Pocket Admission Book–contains blank admit forms $4.00

1-883205-18-2 How to be a Truly Excellent Junior Medical Student–Lederman $12.00

U.S. Public Health Service and other federal agencies

1-883205-32-8 Clinician's Handbook of Preventive Services, 2nd ed.–USPHS $20.00

1-883205-13-1 Guide to Clinical Preventive Services, 2nd ed.–United States Preventive Services Task Force $24.00

1-883205-42-5 The JNC VI Report on Prevention, Detection, Evaluation, and Treatment of High Blood Pressure–NIH $8.95

1-883205-33-6 Health Information for International Travel 1996-97–CDC $14.95

1-883205-45-X 1998 Guidelines for Treatment of Sexually Transmitted Diseases–CDC $7.95

ORDER FORM

In addition to your address, please include an e-mail or phone number so that we might contact you with any questions about your order.

Name: _____

Address: _____

City, State, Zip: _____

Daytime phone/e-mail: _____

❏ Personal Check
❏ Credit Card (circle one):   Visa   Mastercard   Amex   Discover

Card Number _____

Expiration _____

Signature _____

Title	ISBN	Quantity	Price
		Tax 5.75% D.C.	
		S&H (see below)	
		Total	

Sales Tax 5.75% in Washington D.C.

Shipping charges are $5.00 for the first book, $.50 for each additional in the 48 continental states. Please call for other rates.

Please send your order to: Reiter's Scientific & Professional Books, 2021 K Street, N.W., Washington, D.C. 20006.

Information & ordering: 202-223-3327.

Toll free: 800-591-2713. Fax: 202-296-9103.

E-mail inquiries to: books@reiters.com or visit us on the web at www.medicalpublishing.com.

Title List from International Medical Publishing

ISBN — Title — Author — Price

Intern Pocket Survival Guides

0-9634063-0-2 The Intern Pocket Survival Guide–Masterson $7.50
0-9634063-1-0 The CCU Intern Pocket Survival Guide–Masterson/Rothenhaus $7.50
0-9634063-2-9 The ER Intern Pocket Survival Guide–Rothenhaus/Masterson $7.50
0-9634063-3-7 The ICU Intern Pocket Survival Guide–
    Masterson/Rothenhaus/Tenner $7.50
0-9634063-5-3 The Surgical Intern Pocket Survival Guide–Chamberlain $7.50
0-9634063-9-6 The Oncology Intern Pocket Survival Guide–
    Tenner/Masterson/Rollhauser $7.50

Emergency Handbooks

0-9634063-8-8 The EKG Pocket Survival Guide–International Medical
    Publishing $6.00
1-883205-16-6 The ACLS Pocket Survival Guide–International Medical
    Publishing $6.00
1-883205-19-0 The PALS Pocket Survival Guide–International Medical
    Publishing $6.00
1-883205-46-8 The Pocket Guide to Emergency and Disability Scores $6.00
1-883205-20-4 First Aid–Bureau of Mines $6.25

Clinical Practice Handbooks

1-883205-44-1 Pocketful of Prevention–Masterson $7.50
1-883205-39-5 The Gastroenterology Resident Pocket Survival Guide $9.95

Medical Student Titles

0-9634063-6-1 The Pocket Guide to Eponyms and Subtle Signs of Disease–
    Tenner/Masterson $7.50
0-9634063-4-5 The Intern Pocket Admission Book–contains blank admit forms $4.00
1-883205-18-2 How to be a Truly Excellent Junior Medical Student–Lederman $12.00

U.S. Public Health Service and other federal agencies

1-883205-32-8 Clinician's Handbook of Preventive Services, 2nd ed.–USPHS $20.00
1-883205-13-1 Guide to Clinical Preventive Services, 2nd ed.–United States
    Preventive Services Task Force $24.00
1-883205-42-5 The JNC VI Report on Prevention, Detection, Evaluation, and
    Treatment of High Blood Pressure–NIH $8.95
1-883205-33-6 Health Information for International Travel 1996-97–CDC $14.95
1-883205-45-X 1998 Guidelines for Treatment of Sexually Transmitted
    Diseases–CDC $7.95

ORDER FORM

In addition to your address, please include an e-mail or phone number so that we might contact you with any questions about your order.

Name: _____

Address: _____

City, State, Zip: _____

Daytime phone/e-mail: _____

❑ Personal Check
❑ Credit Card (circle one): Visa   Mastercard   Amex   Discover

Card Number _____

Expiration _____

Signature _____

Title	ISBN	Quantity	Price
		Tax 5.75% D.C.	
		S&H (see below)	
		Total	

Sales Tax 5.75% in Washington D.C.

Shipping charges are $5.00 for the first book, $.50 for each additional in the 48 continental states. Please call for other rates.

Please send your order to: Reiter's Scientific & Professional Books, 2021 K Street, N.W., Washington, D.C. 20006.

Information & ordering: 202-223-3327.
Toll free: 800-591-2713. Fax: 202-296-9103.

E-mail inquiries to: books@reiters.com or visit us on the web at www.medicalpublishing.com.

Title List from International Medical Publishing

ISBN — Title — Author — Price

Intern Pocket Survival Guides

0-9634063-0-2 The Intern Pocket Survival Guide–Masterson $7.50
0-9634063-1-0 The CCU Intern Pocket Survival Guide–Masterson/Rothenhaus $7.50
0-9634063-2-9 The ER Intern Pocket Survival Guide–Rothenhaus/Masterson $7.50
0-9634063-3-7 The ICU Intern Pocket Survival Guide–
Masterson/Rothenhaus/Tenner $7.50
0-9634063-5-3 The Surgical Intern Pocket Survival Guide–Chamberlain $7.50
0-9634063-9-6 The Oncology Intern Pocket Survival Guide–
Tenner/Masterson/Rollhauser $7.50

Emergency Handbooks

0-9634063-8-8 The EKG Pocket Survival Guide–International Medical
Publishing $6.00
1-883205-16-6 The ACLS Pocket Survival Guide–International Medical
Publishing $6.00
1-883205-19-0 The PALS Pocket Survival Guide–International Medical
Publishing $6.00
1-883205-46-8 The Pocket Guide to Emergency and Disability Scores $6.00
1-883205-20-4 First Aid–Bureau of Mines $6.25

Clinical Practice Handbooks

1-883205-44-1 Pocketful of Prevention–Masterson $7.50
1-883205-39-5 The Gastroenterology Resident Pocket Survival Guide $9.95

Medical Student Titles

0-9634063-6-1 The Pocket Guide to Eponyms and Subtle Signs of Disease–
Tenner/Masterson $7.50
0-9634063-4-5 The Intern Pocket Admission Book–contains blank admit forms $4.00
1-883205-18-2 How to be a Truly Excellent Junior Medical Student–Lederman $12.00

U.S. Public Health Service and other federal agencies

1-883205-32-8 Clinician's Handbook of Preventive Services, 2nd ed.–USPHS $20.00
1-883205-13-1 Guide to Clinical Preventive Services, 2nd ed.–United States
Preventive Services Task Force $24.00
1-883205-42-5 The JNC VI Report on Prevention, Detection, Evaluation, and
Treatment of High Blood Pressure–NIH $8.95
1-883205-33-6 Health Information for International Travel 1996-97–CDC $14.95
1-883205-45-X 1998 Guidelines for Treatment of Sexually Transmitted
Diseases–CDC $7.95

ORDER FORM

In addition to your address, please include an e-mail or phone number so that we might contact you with any questions about your order.

Name: _____

Address: _____

City, State, Zip: _____

Daytime phone/e-mail: _____

❑ Personal Check
❑ Credit Card (circle one):   Visa   Mastercard   Amex   Discover

Card Number _____

Expiration _____

Signature _____

Title	ISBN	Quantity	Price
		Tax 5.75% D.C.	
		S&H (see below)	
		Total	

Sales Tax 5.75% in Washington D.C.

Shipping charges are $5.00 for the first book, $.50 for each additional in the 48 continental states. Please call for other rates.

Please send your order to: Reiter's Scientific & Professional Books, 2021 K Street, N.W., Washington, D.C. 20006.

Information & ordering: 202-223-3327.
Toll free: 800-591-2713. Fax: 202-296-9103.

E-mail inquiries to: books@reiters.com or visit us on the web at www.medicalpublishing.com.

REGISTRATION

To sign up for updates, errata, more books by this aurthor or in the series, please provide the following information. Include your e-mail address only if International Medical Publishing can include you on their e-mail mailing list.

Name _____

Address _____

City, State, Zip _____

e-mail _____

comments _____

_____

mail to

      International Medical Publishing
      Attn: RPSG
      PO Box 479
      McLean, VA 22101-0479

Or fax to 703-734-8987

Or visit www.medicalpublishing.com

Get Online

Find the Gastroenterology Resident Pocket
Survival Guide online at:
- www.medicalpublishing.com

International Medical Publishing also publishes
resources for people with chronic medical
conditions.

Find patient health calendars online at:
- www.diabetescalendar.com - the Day-by-Day
  Diabetes Calendar
- www.dialysiscalendar.com - the Day-by-Day
  Dialysis Calendar
- www.hivcalendar.com - the Day-by-Day HIV
  Calendar

Resources for people with end stage renal disease
can be found at:
- www.dialysisfinder.com

NOTES

NOTES

NOTES

NOTES

NOTES

NOTES

NOTES

NOTES